Karl Holubar • Stella Fatović-Ferenčić • Gerd Plewig

Looking at Eyes and Faces

Looking at Eyes and Faces

Ophthalmologic water-colours drawn largely by physician-artists
Vienna late 18th and 19th centuries

Karl Holubar, Vienna
Stella Fatović-Ferenčić, Zagreb
Gerd Plewig, Munich

with a panel of contributors

Austrian Academy of Sciences Press
Vienna 2006

From the Department of History of Medicine (Center of Public Health), Medical University of Vienna, Vienna, Austria (K.H.) and the Max and Margareta Wolf Library for the History of Dermatology.

the Croatian Academy of Sciences and Arts, Department for History
and Philosophy of Science, Division for the History of Medical Sciences, Zagreb, Croatia (S.F.F.) and

the Department of Dermatology, Ludwig-Maximilian-University, Munich, Germany (G.P.)

Published in Austria by the
Austrian Academy of Sciences Press
A-1010 Vienna, Dr.-Ignaz-Seipel-Platz 2

ISBN 13: 978-3-7001-3667-5
ISBN 10: 3-7001-3667-6

http://hw.oeaw.ac.at/3667-5
http://verlag.oeaw.ac.at

also under the auspices of the
Croatian Academy of Sciences and Arts

and the
European Society for the History of Dermatology and Venereology
(ESHDV), Paris

Supported by the Austrian National Bank

British Library Cataloguing in Publication data.
A Catalogue record of this book is available from the British Library.

Printed and bound in Austria by „agensketterl" Druckerei GmbH,
A-3001 Mauerbach

Table of Contents

Acknowledgements
Brigitte Maurer, Institute for the History of Medicine, Medical University of Vienna, Vienna, Austria
Agnes Loessl, Archives of the University of Vienna, Vienna, Austria
Verwaltungsarchiv, Staatsarchiv (Federal Archives of the Republic of Austria), Vienna, Austria
Anke Schaening MA, Sigrid Eyb-Green MA, Academy of Fine Arts, Vienna, Austria
Special thanks go to Messrs. Rudolf Nauš, from the printers company "agensketterl", and to Hannes Weinberger from the Austrian Academy's editorial division for their unending patience and diligence.

Explanatory remarks by the principal authors (K.H., S.F.F., G.P.)

This book has been prepared within the frame-work of an inter-academy project Iconography in Medicine, of the Austrian and Croatian Academies of Sciences.
A previous volume, entitled Skin in Water Colours, by the same principal authors appeared at Blackwells, Berlin-Vienna, 2003.
The following gallery of pictures (drawings, gouaches, prints), is a random, but close to complete selection, taken from the files of the Vienna Institute where the images are kept since they were donated by the (then 1st) Department of Ophthalmology, University of Vienna, mainly in the mid-seventies of the 20th century.
The individual pictures were originally entered into the departmental collections during the 19th century, the oldest dated 1782. Numbers were arbitrary and consist, at times, of letters and numbers. No retrograde identification of the date is possible unless the painters had done so. Most but not all were made by physicians and sent to the department or to Vienna from abroad, for diagnostic and/or therapeutic suggestions or for illustrating the patients' history. Few pictures had letters enclosed, which did not however contain specific information except relations to traumas.
For the above reasons we do not include text fragments from such letters or facsimilia (gothic, at times badly legible or illegible hand written texts, in old flowery German). Some of the pictures have previously been published, e.g., prints of GJ Beer in his late 18th and early 19th century book editions, others, individually, e.g., in the bicentennial volume of the Vienna Institute in 1985. No comparable comprehensive edition, as is this one, has ever been undertaken.
Our intention simply was, to present hand made illustrations from up to 200 years ago and have various medical specialists, ophthalmologists in the first place, give their immediate impressions.
We want to emphasize how the eye, the hand, and the brain of a talented physician can prove dexterity and talent in several fields. GJ Beer is a master example because he was an eminent eye surgeon, clinician, and painter. Much like Carl von Rzehaczek our hero from skin paintings as presented in our last book (Skin in Water Colours) who demonstrated his own skill, first, as a painter for Hebra, thereafter as a professor of surgery and head of department at the University of Graz, Austria, and as a sculptor once he had retired from his professorial position.
The sequence of pictures in the book is arbitrary and made so as to provide some of the spectacular paintings to several colleagues equally.
The individual size of the drawings, water colors, gouaches, varied from slightly bigger than natural size of an eye or a pupilla to 35 times 25 cm. Reproduction format was adjusted for practical (and cost) reasons.
Spelling (English/American) and style of English of the individual authors was left unchanged.
Devoted to the Memory of (Dr.) Max Wolf (1892–1990) and his wife Margareta Langer-Wolf (1902–2002), Vienna and New York City.

our skill in language. Wilkinson's chapter lifts us to a higher level of expression, with enchanting stories of word origins for both Ophthalmology and all of medicine. We learn of couching, a surgical treatment for cataracts devised 3,000 years ago by an itinerant Indian doctor. A needle is inserted to push the opaque lens down out of the line of sight, providing instant cure for the common condition making the patient see things as through a cataract of rushing water. We also learned that retina is simply a Greek word for a net, in this case a postage stamp web of cones and rods. The derivation of pupil is entrancing, the Latin word for doll; i.e., what we see is reflected off the cornea of our patient as a diminutive image of our own self.

Another valuable chapter concerns the eye in literature. References include the 13th chapter of James Joyce's Ulysses, concerning our organ of non-verbal sexual communication. Blindness as a punishment and the evil eye are both common in mythology and fairy tales. The eye is often the symbol of God in paintings, and its homophone indicates it is also the symbol for man, i.e., I. The eye is everywhere from the Greek hero, Argus, with his 100 eyes, to the colorful eyes in the Peacock's tail and butterfly wings.

Another chapter concerns the interplay of visual images and the brain in the perception of beauty in virtually all fields ranging from mathematics to sculpture. Here, the physiology of Gestalt comes into play as art works show a pleasing degree of order and complexity. The eye makes a whole from all of the parts, and also enables us to gain perspective. From the evolutionary standpoint, the eye has determined pattern recognition, distinguishing what one can eat from what can eat you.

A separate chapter dwells on the visual aspect of signs and symbols in communication. The eye permits communication by gestures mimic, looks and garments. All of these overlay the spoken word. Thus, we may see more than we hear. In addition, the eyes may express moods, astonishment, boldness, indifference, and even intimidation.

Finally, the authors have a critique on the ethics of medical imagery. They decline to publish a gruesome copper print of the severed head of a syphilitic prostitute. As physicians, we should treat the dead humanely, and not exploit them as icons of sensationalism; nor should we ever forget that medicine remains a humanity. We need an all abiding empathy and compassion. We must never leave the patient alone with NMR shadows, x-ray images, and cold indifferent laboratory numbers. Rejoice or weep with your patients, but never abandon them. All of us will come to the day when our eye will close forever more. Only then are we relieved of duty to our fellow man.

You have in your hands a masterpiece created by three erudite medical historians: Karl Holubar, Stella Fatović-Ferenčić and Gerd Plewig. Enjoy it.

Looking back into the Beer-Jaeger Family

Jan Odorich Abel
Ophthalmologist and seventh generation descendant

There always has to be one person to start a family tradition. At the beginning of this family tradition, which means to become an eye specialist, stands Georg Joseph Beer (1763–1821) (Fig.1). He started his medical career of becoming a surgeon. It was not easy for him to become an ophthalmologist, but he struggled against all odds at the time and finally, he was and still is, known for founding the first university department of ophthalmology located in the Vienna General Hospital.

Georg Joseph Beer was very popular at the time and many of well known personalities of the time consulted him. Although he treated many wealthy people, he always cared for the poor.

One of Beer's assistants was Friedrich Christoph Jaeger von Jaxtthal (1784–1871). He got to know George Joseph Beer through his brother Carl. Carl Jaeger von Jaxtthal lived in Kirchberg, Germany, and came to Vienna to study medicine. Here he met Beer and some years later, Carl's brother Friedrich Christoph, followed Carl, to improve his skills as an eye specialist. He became acquainted with the Beer family.

During the attack of Napoleon on Vienna, the house, where Beer lived and had his surgery, was bombed and someone had to rescue the patients and the daughter Therese Beer. Therese, who was 11 years old at that time, had typhoid fever and had to stay in bed. Friedrich Christoph Jaeger von Jaxtthal carried Therese down the stairs into the sub basement as well as some of the patients. No one of the Beer family or the patients was injured. Because of rescuing his one and only daughter, Beer looked at Friedrich Christoph as member of the family. Therese survived the infection.

Many years later, Therese Beer and Friedrich Christoph Jaeger von Jaxtthal got married on the 15th of January 1815. At that time, Jaeger was chief physician of the military medical academy, the Josephinum, and was consulted regularly by Metternich, Austria's chancellor. Although Jaeger was very successful, he never held a chair in Vienna, because he did not want to go to Budapest, which would have been the academic prerequisite to get a professorship in Vienna, as customary in many countries.

Friedrich Christoph Jaeger von Jaxtthal and Therese had four children. One of them, Eduard Jaeger von Jaxtthal (1818–1884), got in touch with patients at a very early age. His father took him along into the surgery theaters and Eduard was allowed to give his father a helping hand during examinations and operations. His passion for medicine soon became his profession and he became a famous eye specialist. Eduard eventually was appointed (founder)-chairman and professor of the 2nd University Department at Vienna. The fame of Eduard Jaeger von Jaxtthal was well-founded by his adaptation of the ophthalmoscope to examine the fundus of the eye, an instrument devised by Helmholtz in 1851. He later published the first ophthalmoscopic atlas.

Eduard and his wife Marie Josepha Augusta, who died young, had two children. Their son Carl became a qualified engineer. The daughter, Marie Christine Augusta, got married to Dr. Karl Dengg, who was a lawyer. They had three children. One of their daughters was Friedericke Dengg, who married Professor Othenio Abel. Othenio Abel and Louis Dollo are known for founding the department of palaeobiology of Vienna University.

Othenio Abel and his wife had two children. Their son was Dr. Wolfgang Abel, my father. He was an anthropologist and was a lecturer at the University in Berlin.

At this time, my own story begins. I grew up in Upper Austria, in the country side. But because of my family, talking about life in academia, I conceived the idea of an academic education. At the age of 16, I knew exactly what kind of profession I would like to go in for: an ophthalmologist. I never intended to become a university lecturer. Of course, I knew I needed a good education, so I went to Vienna and started medical school. As I finished my studies at the University of Vienna, I went through the training at the 2nd University Department of Ophthalmology under Professors Josef Böck and Hans Slezak. After some time I was promoted to senior physician and soon I wondered, where I should go from now on. All of a sudden, I got the chance to fulfill my dream of having my own surgery in a small town. In the town of Baden, south of Vienna, my dream really came true. I moved there with my family. For 30 years I am working as an eye specialist and it was always my aim to help every patient, who needs help. By now, I teach young doctors, just as Beer did, and it is good to know that the knowledge I gained, goes on.

Fig. 1
Georg Joseph Beer 1763–1821

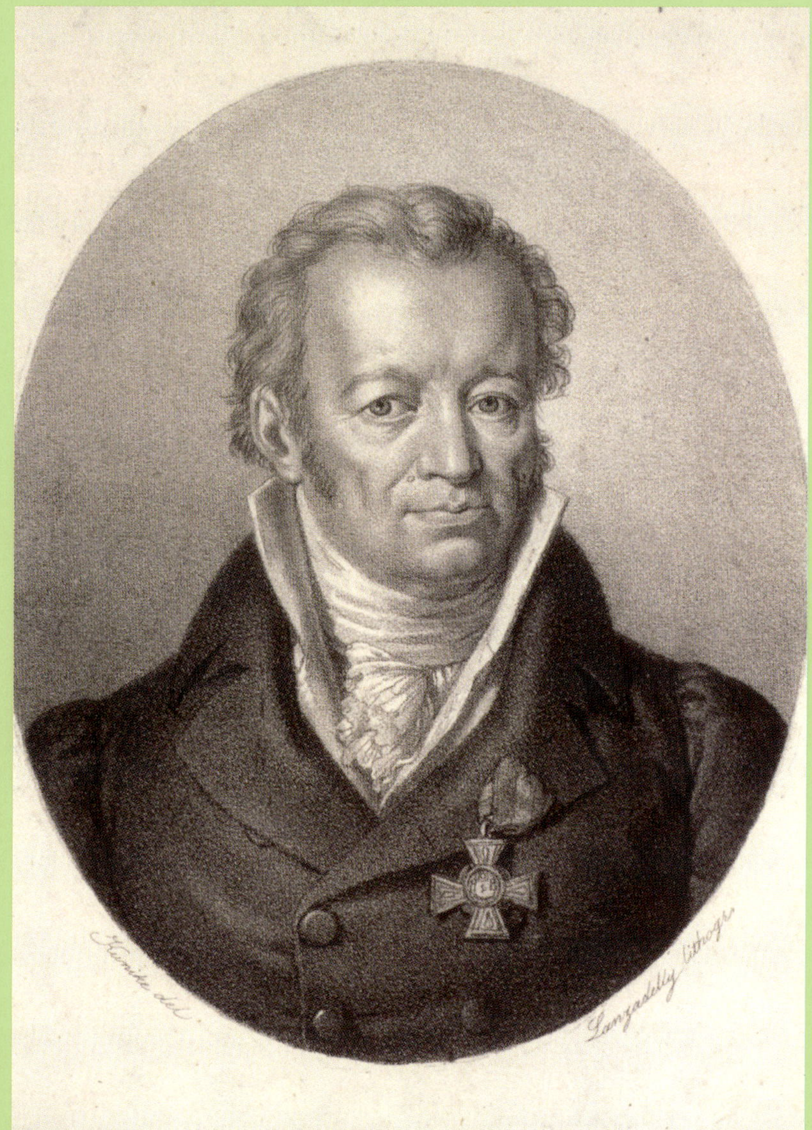
Kunike del
Lanzedelly lithogr.

The Vienna School of Ophthalmology and its Roots

Karl Holubar and Stella Fatović-Ferenčić

Vienna has a university since 1365. Between 1785 and 1874 a separate medico-surgical military academy existed; since 2004 there is a Medical University of Vienna. In the field of medicine, international fame was achieved only after Gerard van Swieten's (1700–1772) reforms under Empress Maria Theresa (1717–1780). Surgery received its decisive stimulus by her son, Joseph II (1741–1790), who took as an example the French Académie Royale de Chirurgie in Paris and set up a military medical academy in his own capital city. This institution soon reached international rank. By 1804 it even had a special practical training school for surgeons. Obviously, ophthalmologic surgery flourished, since next to surgical doctorates also master's degrees in ophthalmology were conferred to its élèves. Any historical summary of the development of a school for eye diseases and their treatment must start at this point of time.

The Foundation of the Josephine Academy (Josephinum)

For more than three centuries, the area between Alser Strasse and Währinger Strasse, harbours the facilities of what became the university hospital and the central military hospital of the city of Vienna. At the far end, along the eastern side of this complex, the Schola Anatomico Medico-Chirurgica (as inscribed on the buiding), or, in full, Academia caesareo-regia Iosephina Medico-chirurgica Vindobonensis, the Josephinum as referred to colloquially, is located (Fig. 2). "Within its walls, history can be experienced" reads the Festschrift[1, p.6] on occasion of the bicentennial of the foundation, and Claudio Magris wrote[2, ch.16, p.203] "... l'antica accademia voluta da Giuseppe II per i suoi chirurghi militari, dalla quale è uscita la grande scuola clinica viennese". After the dismemberment of the old empire and the dissolution of the imperial army, the Institute for the History of Medicine of the University of Vienna was housed there and permitted to take over the heritage, and thrive in the genius loci[3,4]. Romeo Seligmann (1808–1892), the first professor of this discipline in Vienna[5] was eager already 150 years ago to take into possession the Josephine Library and the Florentine anatomical waxes, something only his second successor, Max Neuburger (1868–1955) could achieve. Magris again[2, p.204] "questo museo delle cere non è un museo degli orrori, perche la verità rende liberi e la conoscenza della materia, che noi siamo, la rende degna d'amore". This tesoro nazionale italiano-austriaco is proudly displayed within its halls for more than two hundred years to the present day.

When the Josephine military academy was formally inaugurated on Monday 7th November 1785[1,6], one year after the adjoining poor-house and veterans' hospital had been streamlined and opened as a general and university hospital, this institution could be seen as the embodiment of the ideas of a strong willed sovereign and a talented medical administrator acting in tandem: Joseph II, impartial, open to the ideas of enlightenment with a zest to reform his country and its institutions, and Giovanni Alessandro Brambilla (1728–1800), counsellor and advisor, slightly older than the monarch, and playing a role not dissimilar to the one Gerard van Swieten had played for Joseph's mother. Modelled after the Académie Royale de Chirurgie (1731) in Paris, it was designed to educate military surgeons and confer academic status to them, thereby creating a parallel medical establishment side by side with the doctores graduating from the university medical school. A higher two-year course leading to a master's or a doctoral degree, and a lower 6-months' course were offered. The former for selected military personnel with previous experience and the latter for talented freshmen. Five professores ordinarii were appointed to form the academy's staff of teachers (i) for anatomy and physiology including geometry and physics, Wilhelm Böcking (1742–1804), (ii) for general pathology, therapy and hygiene, Heinrich Streit (1745–1821), (iii) for surgery, obstetrics and forensic medicine, Johann Hunczovsky (1752–1798), (iv) for internal medicine (in modern parlance), Joseph Gabriel von Gabriely (1744–1806), and (v) for botanic, chemistry and pharmacology, Joseph Plenck (1735–1807). Two of these professors, Joseph Plenck and Johann Hunczovsky, were outstanding teachers and authors (viz. the former's treatise of 1776 on skin diseases, which served as the basis of Robert Willan's (1757–1812) epochal classification). Two other men served right from the opening of the Josephinum, not as professors yet: Anton Beinl von Bienenburg (1749–1820) as prosector, and Johann Adam Schmidt (1759–1809) as Brambilla's secretary. The latter, later on professor for pathology and therapy, ophthalmology and pharmacology, created the terms pharmacognosy and pharmacodynamics. He was Ludwig van Beethoven's physician, to whom the master gratefully dedicated so nicely the Trio op.#38. Schmidt became one of the first pupils of Joseph Barth (1745–1818).

Joseph II died in 1790 and his brainchild the Josephinum became an orphan. Shortly thereafter, Brambilla retired in 1795, and died in 1800. First criticisms were uttered and reforms were carried out. The imbroglio caused by the French revolution and by the upcoming Napoleonic era did not leave the Josephinum unaffected. The state was formally transformed and the Holy Roman Empire became the heritable Empire of Austria. Battered by Napoleon, the country was shifted around in Central Europe geo-politically, cut off from the sea and deprived of essential provinces; state bankruptcy had to be declared and only after two decades a sort of status quo ante and stability, could be achieved. No wonder that an institution which was to serve the military in the first place, was a prime victim of such fundamental changes. Eventually, in 1820, the Josephinum was closed temporarily for the first time to be reformed and reopened only two years later. It must be emphasized however, that the establishment of this military medical school, as we would call it today, had important formative influence on the development of surgery, ophthalmology and obstetrics. Midwifery was drifting into the hands of trained obstetricians, eye surgeons were not just educated in barbers' shops, nor were surgeons in general. The army medical corps now consisted of, we would say today, board certified men. The first special institute to practically train surgeons, was opened at the Josephinum in 1804 in the midst of all the political turmoil, and served as a role model for the opening of a similar postgraduate training school by the university of Vienna.

In 1848, again, the purpose of the Josephine academy came under doubt and plans to merge it with the university were made. It was once more closed for some years and reorganized, to be reopened again in 1852 and under different auspices in 1854, to be finally shut down on 16th July 1874 when the medical and surgical students' curricula were unified. Many celebrities had been on the staff in the Josephinum's last period[7]. In the following 40-odd years, ad finem imperii in 1918, the Josephinum just served as a sort of postgraduate institute for military doctors. After World War I, Karel Frederik Wenckebach (1864–1940), a Dutch, and head of the Department of Internal Medicine I, at Vienna University, proposed to house History of Medicine in the building of the Josephinum, a proposal which was accepted and enacted by the faculty[(3,4)]. Max Neuburger moved in and hereby realized his and his two predecessors' dreams: to be in charge of the famous library, the equally famous anatomical waxes and, after all, to have a seat in a historically dignified building.

The Formal Development of the Vienna School of Ophthalmology

This elaboration first poses a semantic problem: What is a school?
Where there is a teacher (master) and where there are pupils?
Where there is a teacher with an academic appointment?
a docent (lecturer)
a professor

Where there is a big hospital providing enough patients for teaching
and a master utilizing these provisions?

Where there is a university, i.e., a public academic institution with teachers who carry an academic appointment and who have a filiation of pupils emerging from this place?

To elaborate in detail on these questions would be beyond the scope of this chapter. We have addressed it sometime ago with regard to dermatology[(8)]. Still another question is left for consideration, namely, what is a chair (cattedra)? Do only professors have a chair or also holders of a lower academic qualification (docentes). In this context we will just refer to professorships and university schools existing over longer periods (decades or more). Eduardo Midena in his bicentennial Festschrift in Padua[(9)] wrote, that the first two professorships of ophthalmology were erected in Paris and in Vienna in the third quarter of the Settecento. Ovio[(10)] writes the same, giving 1765 and 1773 as years of establishment in either city, Hirsch[(11)], and Hirschberg[(12)] mention 1762 for Paris; for Vienna 1773 is certain. On the other hand, Manché of Malta, Clinica oculistica 1893, p.1433, as quoted by

Hirschberg,[12,p.489, footnote] wrote: "La prima Catedra di Ottalmologia, in tutte le università del mondo venne istituta a Vienna e pel primo occupata da un maltese")

The archives in Vienna[13a] display the appointment of Joseph Barth (1745-1818) of Malta, as öffentlicher Lehrer (in German) on 23rd October 1773. The subsequent year he was referred to as "... Barth Professor Anatomiae et oculorum morborum ac consiliarius declaratur ..." which makes certain that the German phrase "öffentlicher Lehrer" meant the same as "Professor". (Fig. 3, a b). There was no parallel establishment of a university department of eye diseases with this professorship at the time.

Few years afterwards, Pietro Antonio dalla Bona in Padua, was appointed by the senate of the Serenissima as professor morborum artificum, puerorum et oculorum, on 24th September 1785, effective 1st October of that year (The professorship became obsolete when the Serenissima fell in 1797 and the university was closed)[9]. Barth in Vienna retired from his chair in 1791 and was succeeded by Georg Prochaska (1749-1820). Next to him, Johann Adam Schmidt (1759-1809) at the Josephinum, was appointed professor in 1795 (imperial manuproprio by Francis I., dated Laxenburg 18th June 1795)[13b]. Eye diseases were included in this appointment "if time allows" as indicated in the decree of the Hofkriegsrath dated 1st September 1796[13c]. His teaching comprised pathology, therapy, pharmacology and prescriptions, and "if time allows", eye diseases and venereal diseases. Eventually, in this file of ophthalmologists in academia in Vienna, Georg Joseph Beer (1763-1821) followed as professor in 1812.

So far the sequence of ordination of the first professors for (better, also for) eye diseases and eye surgery. There were no separate university departments of ophthalmology at any of these places, and not at the Josephinum in Vienna at the time. This notwithstanding, all these gentlemen had their small private clinics and operated also in public or in military hospitals. In 1812 eventually, the imperial government in Vienna decided to establish a university department for eye diseases, to be headed by Georg Joseph Beer, who had been appointed professor for this field already in March[14], and who started his lectures in April of that year[7 p.82]. The department of Beer appears to be the oldest continually existing and the oldest university department of the specialty. Suffice it to say that the term ophthalmology was proposed by Karl Himly (1722-1837) in 1801, and universally adopted later in the 19th century. Johann Adam Schmidt, in the first article of the first volume of the Ophthalmologische Bibliothek[15], still considers the terms of ophthalmonosology and ophthalmiatry as alternatives (such terminological questions are discussed elsewhere[16]).

Let us now return to Vienna and the period before Barth was appointed in 1773. First attention to the teaching of eye diseases and their therapy was given in Vienna by Gerard van Swieten (1700-1772), as much as by the imperial court. Baron Michael Johann Wenzel, was invited to treat patients and perform model operations. He charged considerable honoraria. Eventually, Joseph Barth was appointed professor of anatomy and eye diseases, including eye operations. He trained in eye surgery in Paris but neither Lesky[7] nor

Hirschberg[12] mention when. Joseph II had a contract made with him in 1790, with the provision to train two other physicians, in turn for his own training abroad. One of these two pupils was Johann Adam Schmidt (1759–1809)*, the other Barth's prosector Johann Ehrenritter (who died soon thereafter). Barth's personal profile is described differently in the literature, in high praise by his pupil Johann Adam Schmidt, much more critically, e.g., by Hirschberg. In any case, he was the first professor in the field in Vienna and he employed the young Georg Joseph Beer as a painter and drawer while he still was a medical student. The earliest water colour in our files is dated 1785 when Beer was a student and 22 years old. Narrow-mindedly, Barth did not make his expertise in the field of ophthalmology available to his amanuensis Beer (as Lesky called him[7 p.80]). Beer had to gather experience on his own. He ran an ophthalmologic practice, later also a public ambulance for the poor. Barth retired 1791 and was followed by Georg Prochaska (1749–1820), an anatomist and professor also for eye diseases, from Prague (imperial manuproprio by Leopold II. dated 19th September 1791[13b]). Prochaska also taught ophthalmology and he jealously tried to ward off Beer's attempts to have an eye department established. In the Salzburger medizinisch-chirurgische Zeitung 1798[17, vol 4 p.44-48]. Beer published a proposal to establish an eye clinic consisting of five rooms, two with four beds, one for men, one for women, who cannot pay by themselves for treatment, and two rooms with two beds each, for paying patients. The fifth room should be used for lectures. Beer also proposed two courses of lectures per year, given by himself of five months duration each, four days a week, 11–12 AM, followed by clinical rounds 12 noon to 1 PM on the same days. The lecture room should hold a pertinent library. Only students who had finished medical school were to be admitted and costs would be 13 guilders 20 crowns per course. His own treatise on diseases of the eye was to serve as a textbook. Thoughtful and detailed indeed. But, Beer did not succeed with his efforts, the government turned it down.

Unfortunately, Johann Adam Schmidt died in 1809 and thereby, a reduction of activities in the discipline-to-be, took place. Beer's perseverance eventually got him the rank of professor extraordinary in the spring of 1812 (imperial resolution of 23rd March 1812), an appointment which was followed by the decree to establish a university department on 26th November of the same year[14]. Beer became professor ordinarius in 1818. He died in 1821 and was followed by Anton Rosas (1791–1855).

During the first decade of the century, Schmidt in the Josephinum and Beer (still without academic appointment) were engaged in therapeutic discussions, e.g., as to the preferred method of cataract operations and iridectomy. After Schmidt's demise, Beer was the undisputed leader of the Vienna School, Anton Rosas and Friedrich Jaeger (1784–1872) growing up. Beer became sick in his latest period in office and Jaeger, who had become

---

* J.A. Schmidt was Ludwig van Beethoven's physician to whom the master dedicated Trio op.# 38 in B Flat Major, developed from Septetto op.# 20, set "easily" so as to enable Schmidt to play it with his family. The dedication on Page one of the piano part begins" Monsieur! Je sens parfaitement bien, que la Célébrité de Votre nom, ainsi que l'amitié dont Vous m'honorez exigeroit de moi la dédicace d'un bien plus important ouvrage». and it ends «... Vous reconnoissez toute la vivacité et la cordialité de mes sentiments. Louis van Beethoven.»

his son-in-law was expected to succeed him, a situation as it re-appeared in dermatology decades later, when Ferdinand Hebra's (1816–1880) son-in-law Moriz Kaposi (1837–1902) did aspire to, and finally achieve, to follow his father-in-law in office.

At this point of time, Budapest and Padua universities were to be provided with a suitable candidate each, for the ophthalmologic chairs. Rosas went to Italy, to hold the chair for two years in the re-opened university in Padua (1819). Jaeger, however, refused to leave Vienna to the chagrin of the almighty ministerial director, Baron Andreas Joseph Stifft (1760–1836). When Beer finally died in 1821, it was Rosas to be entrusted and called back from Padua, and Jaeger had to sit it out till he made it for the chair in the Josephinum which he held until 1848. Jaeger did not write much, rather had his views expressed by his pupils. He is described as an extremely skilful (eye) surgeon, an ability which earned him fame throughout Europe, including by the princely houses from Hanover to Constantinople, as Lesky has it[7, p. 88].

The existence of a military medical school (Josephinum) in parallel to the university, created a competition within medical academia in Vienna, especially so because the Allgemeine Krankenhaus (general hospital, civil) and the Garnisons-Spital (garrison hospital, military) were located in physical proximity within the same architectural complex. This academic competition was enhanced when second chairs of surgery and internal medicine (1842 and 1849) were established. In the field of specialty disciplines, circumstances were not much different. Two examples may be given:

Ophthalmology, which had a university department from 1812, and one in the Josephinum from 1826. A second university chair followed in 1883 when the Josephinum was closed already for good.

Dermatology, which had two chairs (skin and syphilis) erected in 1849 and a third in the Josephinum in 1870.

One can easily imagine that potential candidates for these chairs were vieing for one or the other, or moving from one over to the other, the university chairs always being considered more desirable.

As we have seen, Friedrich Jaeger (1784–1872) did not make it to succeed his father-in-law but was eventually appointed to the chair of ophthalmology in the Josephinum which he held for more than 22 years. His most talented pupil was his own son Eduard Jaeger (1818–1884), who became head of a non-university department and only one year before he died became chairman of the newly established second university chair in 1883.

Beer's chair was taken by Rosas as pointed out above, in 1821. After Rosas followed Ferdinand Arlt (1812-1887) in 1856. A jealous competition between the Arlt and Jaeger schools resulted, which dominated the scene of the discipline in Vienna for decades. This notwithstanding, ophthalmology had reached fame in the city, which radiated into France and Germany and other European countries. Most importantly, Albrecht von Greafe must be mentioned, as one of the most prominent pupils of Ferdinand Arlt. The acquaintance of Graefe with both Jaegers established the relation with the emerging German School. In January of 1854 Graefe launched the Archiv für Ophthalmologie, the oldest journal of the field in German, still going strong today. A late 19th century highlight of the achievements in ophthalmology in Vienna was the introduction of cocaine as a local anaesthetic in 1884, by Carl Koller (1857–1944) an outcome of the Freud-Lustgarten-Koller endeavours, i.e., by the Judeo-Viennese Cocaine-Trio. Sigmund Freud jokingly addressed Koller in his letters as Coca-Koller[(18)].

In 1885 eventually, Ernst Fuchs (1851–1930) took the second chair which he held until 1915. He was well known and internationally famous proponent of ophthalmology of the socalled 2nd Medical School of Vienna[(19)].

With regard to publications of the first Vienna School, Beer's Textbook of Ophthalmology (Lehre der Augenkrankheiten) shall be mentioned in the first place. Altogether there are about a dozen texts or editions by Beer between 1792 and 1813/1817[(20)]. The best and most detailed reference to Beer's books is given by Hirschberg, in Graefe's Handbuch der gesamten Augenheilkunde, Engelmann, Leipzig 1911, vol 14, p. 491–534[(12)]. The first edition of Beer's textbook came out in 1792 when the author was 29 years old. Contemporaries criticized him for having copied other authors. Later editions, in 1813 and again 1817, are to be considered exemplary and served as a basis for teaching for Beer and many of his pupils. The drawings of various conditions and of instruments are partly coloured. Seven tables of the 1817 edition depict some 40-odd single eyes displaying various pathological conditions. Of many, no originals exist, others are included in our series; at times, it is difficult to differentiate. The drawings document his artistic talent, a capability also his son-in-law and grandson, i.e., the two Jaegers were graced with. Hirschberg concludes „Beer gehört zu den wenigen Genies die sich spät entwickeln“[(12, p. 518)].

Beer's writings on the history of ophthalmology, i.e., his Bibliotheca ophthalmica are dealt with in the chapter on Ophthalmologische Bibliothek (see below). This text must not be confused with Himly's and Johann Adam Schmidt's periodical having an almost identical title albeit in German.

The visual sense always was believed to be of special importance for a reasonable quality of life, sung by poets, composers and writers. Specialists in eye diseases we find mentioned already by Herodotus and it is no surprise that ophthalmology was to become the first clinical specialty discipline sensu strictiori.

Albrecht von Graefe, in 1851, when reasoning vis-à-vis his mother on his determination to become an ophthalmologist, called the eye das edelste Organ (the most noble organ), and he speaks of its clarity and transparency enabling him to find answers to pathological and

this review referring to Himly. It is not surprising therefore that the preface of volume 1 of the Ophthalmologische Bibliothek expresses the intention to edit a journal of ophthalmology. The preface alludes to the cooperation between the two editors (Himly and Schmidt) in this effort, but it is written by Himly alone, possibly for reasons of proximity of the printers in Braunschweig and Himly's residence in Göttingen and Jena. The pages of the preface are numbered with Roman numerals I-X and dated in Jena, April 1802.

Ophthalmology may be taken as the oldest of the clinical medical specialty disciplines. No wonder then that a specialty journal was edited so early on. This has to be compared with general medical journals, e.g., the Salzburger medizinisch-chirurgische Zeitung which started to appear in 1790, the New England Journal of Medicine in 1812, the Lancet in 1823, Behrend's Syphilidologie in 1839, Cazenave's Annales des maladies de la peau et de la syphilis in 1844, the Wiener medizinische Wochenschrift in 1851, and the Archiv für Ophthalmologie in 1854.

Albrecht von Graefe's editorial, of January 1854, in volume one of the latter journal(1) starts with similar wording as does Himly's half a century earlier(23). Another remarkable fact is that original articles were contained in the Ophthalmologische Bibliothek, right from volume one, at a time, when journal articles frequently referred to original publications elsewhere, or reviewed books and dissertations, presented letters and circulars and notes.

Himly announced that three different genres of papers would be contained in the periodical:
Detailed original papers which should not be a playground of empirics; must be of practical value; and form the basis of theories or deliver results which promise further insights. What a challenge!

Critical referrals to publications pertinent to ophthalmology, out of Germany and her neighbours. All had to be signed, nothing anonymous was permitted.

Short notices, questions, answers, supplements, announcements. It is pointed out that there will be several annual instalments but without any given periodicity. Purposeful entries would be payed for.

The first volume lists four original articles, eight critiques (reviews) and 13 miscellaneous notices.

The first original article is by Johann Adam Schmidt and runs over 44 pages, entitled On ophthalmonosology and ophthalmiatrics as a theory and art. A very thorough if partly

(1) The Archiv für Ophthalmologie was edited at Jeanrenaud's in Berlin. Jeanrenaud was a friend of Graefe's from his years in the French Gymnasium in Berlin. On occasion of a walk in the Prater in Vienna with Friedrich Jaeger, during Graefe's first visit in the city, he was told by his friend about Helmholtz' construction of the ophthalmoscope, as so nicely described in Blida Heynold von Greafe's monography on her grandfather, Stapp, Berlin 1970, ref. 24 p.39

philosophical treatise in which many older and contemporary authors are quoted, viz., Boerhaave, Monro (secundus?), Scarpa, Blumenbach et al. On page 36 it reads: In dieser Zeit lebet nur e i n Mann, der den Genius seiner Zeit überflog ... Joseph Barth ..., a praise, by Schmidt, of his teacher in ophthalmology, and first professor of this discipline in Vienna (1773). The other original articles refer to the Lycée des aveugles in Paris, to ophthalmia in Egypt and to a new method of operating cataracta.

If one looks into the pages of contemporary medical periodicals, e.g., into the aforementioned Salzburger journal[22] in an attempt to finding allusions to newcomers, such as the Ophthalmologische Bibliothek, interesting facts emerge, and proof can be found, that the competition between specialists, professional envy, and jealousy, were rampant then as it is today.

At the time there were no university departments of ophthalmology and no separate chairs of the specialty. Barth was professor of anatomy and ophthalmology including eye surgery but without any public hospital basis. Similarly, Schmidt and Himly were professors also for this field. The time for specialty departments still was to come. For instance, Jean-Louis Alibert, the famous French dermatologist, entrusted in 1801 with the directorship of the Hôpital Saint-Louis in Paris, was no professor at this point of time. But this did not exclude professional chagrin springing up in the pages of contemporary periodicals. In the preface of the Ophthalmologische Bibliothek, volume 1/1, in a footnote, Himly alludes to a controversy with Georg Joseph Beer[22]. This controversy is evident also from the pages of the Salzburger medizinisch-chirurgische Zeitung. Even the latter's editor, Johann Jacob Hartenkeil (1761–1808) comes into play, because he, unintentionally, became the cause of conflict. He had, apparently in good faith, changed the place of mailing of a letter to his journal from Vienna, where Beer lived, to Braunschweig, where Himly was about to edit his Ophthalmologische Bibliothek. Himly seemingly believed that this was some trick by Beer, and Beer assumed that Himly wants to fool him. Eventually, the letters to the editor were certified by notaries (sic!). In regard to this particular facet of the matter, we have it better today, because no journal would accept frequent pros and contras, and most importantly, the delay in publication would take off steam from any such in-fight without substance. Anyway, it is another proof from the scientific world of then, namely, that the respective authors in Europe were quite swift and responsive to make their points, and be it only for procedural details. One would believe that this is only possible in the world of computers. Nay! Even before there was a railway, researchers were quick to react, say, Ritter and Herschel, Blumenbach and Cuvier, Bassi and Schoenlein, to name but a few from the orbit of the sciences of early 19th century.

Without any doubt the Ophthalmologische Bibliothek must be viewed as an early quality publication, very likely of great merit to practitioners and leaders in the field alike. Browsing through the pages, theoretical and philosophical treatises of two hundred years ago teach us a lot: Many thoughts of today were as familiar to our professional forefathers as they are to us.

The Collaboration with the German School

Systematic teaching of ophthalmology in universities started in the 19th century. The same holds for the establishment of university departments in the discipline. Vienna holds a proud tradition in both respects and the First Vienna School of Barth-Beer-Rosas-Arlt had a profound influence in neighbouring countries.

If we consider that Beer's pupils occupied a number of chairs, e.g., Franz Flarer (1791–1850) 1819 in Pavia, Anton von Rosas (1791–1855) 1819 in Padua, Johann Nepomuk Fischer (1777–1847) 1820 in Prague, Friedrich Jaeger (1784–1871) 1826 in the Josephinum in Vienna, to name just a few, the influence of his teachings and writings were guaranteed. Through the Jaegers, and through Ferdinand Arlt, who all three were well acquainted with Albrecht von Graefe (1828–1870), it was ascertained that this rising star of schools of 19th century ophthalmology in Germany was familiar with the perspectives of the Vienna School. The arena of the German language allowed for unhindered exchange of information and Graefe's Archiv für Ophthalmologie (1854) as much as the Deutsche Ophthalmologische Gesellschaft (1857) developed into the central arenas of publication and discussion in Austria and in Germany. No better example can be quoted as Koller's introduction of cocaine into local ophthalmologic anaesthesia in 1884. This discovery was reported instantly in Heidelberg at the above society's meeting only days after the experiments. The presentation was made not by Koller himself, but by Joseph Brettauer (1835–1905), an Austro-Italian oculist from Trieste, because Koller was still in training and only specialists were allowed to participate in the meeting.

At the time when specialty disciplines developed and specialty societies and journals were founded, the common language ensured that concourses for chairs were open to candidates from all corners of the area and specialists, e.g., ophthalmologists or dermatologists or internists were ordinary members of the German societies in the field. There was a circulation of professors between Austria and Germany and the flow of information was easy. The example of Koller or, as outlined in the foregoing chapter, of Graefe and his being told in Vienna about the construction of an ophthalmoscope, may illustrate the situation. Generally it may be said that the political weight of the countries had some reflection also in medicine. In the first half of the 19th century Vienna was the more important centre, in the second half Berlin grew more and more important. German industry dominated chemistry and optics, and the strict and well organized system of German university education bore fruit. By the turn of the 20th century the centre of gravity of medical progress, in ophthalmology and otherwise, had shifted north.

The Vienna School of Ophthalmology in the first half of the 19th century laid the groundwork for the growth of the specialty discipline in Europe. Beer's and Rosas' textbooks, the Jaegers' virtuosity in eye surgery, the refinement of the ophthalmoscope by Eduard Jaeger and his ophthalmoscopic atlas, the first of its kind, were the fruits of the professionalism and erudite scholarship as much as of mutual competition intra muros, on which the region could build.

References

(1) Wyklicky H: Das Josephinum. Biographie eines Hauses. Brandstätter, Wien 1985
(2) Magris C: Danubio. Garzanti, Milano 1986
(3) Neuburger M: Das Institut für Geschichte der Medizin and der k.k. Universität in Wien. Wien klin Wochenschr 1914; 21:566-567
(4) Neuburger M: Das Institut für Geschichte der Medizin an der Universität in Wien. Wien med Wochenschr 1921; 71:70-71
(5) Holubar K: Zur Vorgeschichte der Gründung des medizinhistorischen Lehrstuhles an der Universität Wien (1833-1848/50). Wien med Wochenschr 1990; 140; 441-445
(6) Kirchenberger S: Kaiser Joseph II. als Reformator des österreichischen Militär-Sanitätswesens. Wien 1890
(7) Lesky E: Die Wiener medizinische Schule im 19. Jahrhundert. Böhlau, Graz-Köln, 1965
(8) Marri Malacrida L, Panconesi E, Holubar K: Vincenzio Chiarugi (1759-1820): The academic career of the first professor of skin diseases. Ital Gen Rev Dermatol 1991; 28:129-130
(9) Midena E: 200 Years of ophthalmology. Piccin Padova 1986
(10) Ovio G: Storia dell' oculistica. Ghibaudo, Cuneo 1950
(11) Hirsch A. Biographisches Lexikon der hervorragenden Ärzte aller Zeiten und Völker. Urban & Schwarzenberg, Wien und Leipzig, 1887 vol V, p.241
(12) Hirschberg J: Geschichte der Augenheilkunde. In: Graefe-Saemisch Handbuch der gesamten Augenheilkunde. Engelmann Leipzig, 2nd ed vol XIV
(13) Archives of the University of Vienna and Austrian Federal Archives
(a) Acta facultatis, Archiv der Universität, Vienna 1773 1774
(b) Verwaltungsarchiv 4 Med Wien 131 ex 1790, 179 ex 1791
(c) Kriegsarchiv, Hofkriegsrath 1796
(14) Holubar K: Anton (von) Rosas (1791-1855): On the occasion of the bicentennial of his birth; part I. Wien klin Wochenschr 1991; 103:470-472
(15) Schmidt JA: Ansicht der Ophthalmonosologie und Ophthalmiatrik als Theorie und Kunst im Jahre 1801. Ophthalmologische Bibliothek 1802, vol 1, part 1, p 1-44
(16) Schmidt CC, Holubar K: Von Anatomie bis Andrologie: Zur Entwicklung der medizinischen Fachbezeichnungen. Wien klin Wochenschr 1993; 105:92-93
(17) Beer JG: Nachricht von einem zu errichtenden Klinikum für Augenkrankheiten. Salzb med-chir Zeitg 1798; 4:44-48
(18) Amm M, Holubar K: „Coca Koller"und seine Freunde. Zum 140. Geburtstag des jüdisch-wienerischen Trios: Carl Koller, Sigmund Lustgarten und Sigmund Freud. Wien klin Wochenschr 1997; 109:170-175
(19) Schmidt G: (in press): Das Auge zur Welt: Ernst Fuchs (1851-1930) und die Weltgeltung der Wiener Augenheilkunde um 1900
(20) Wyklicky H: Zur Geschichte der Augenheilkunde in Wien/Ophthalmology in Vienna (German/English) Brandstätter, Vienna 1984
(21) Ophthalmologische Bibliothek, vol 1 part 1, ed Karl Himly and Johann Adam Schmidt, FB Culemann, Braunschweig, 1802; from vol 1 part 2, at F. Frommann, Jena
vol 1, part 1, 1802, p. I-X, and p.VII-VIII, footnote
vol 1, part 1, 1802, p. 1-44 (Schmidt's article)
(22) Salzburger medizinisch-chirurgische Zeitung, ed Hartenkeil JJ, printed at Oberer FX, Salzburg, from 1790 on in, roughly, weekly intervals. The issues were available at all post offices. 54 volumes appeared, four per year.
vol 17, part 1, 1802, p. 58, # 1, 2 January
vol 21, part 1, 1803, p. 63-64, #4, 14 January
vol 22, part 2, 1803, p. 115-123, #33, 25 April
(23) Archiv für Ophthalmologie, 1854, ed von Graefe A, Jeanrenaud, Berlin 1854, vol 1, preface
(24) Graefe, Blida Heynold von: Albrecht von Graefe: Mensch und Umwelt. Stapp, Berlin 1970

Fig. 2
The Imperial Military Medical Academy, the Josephinum, built 1783–1785, by Joseph II (1741–1790). Print after a design by Isidore Canevale. Address: Währinger Strasse 25, A-1090 Vienna IX.

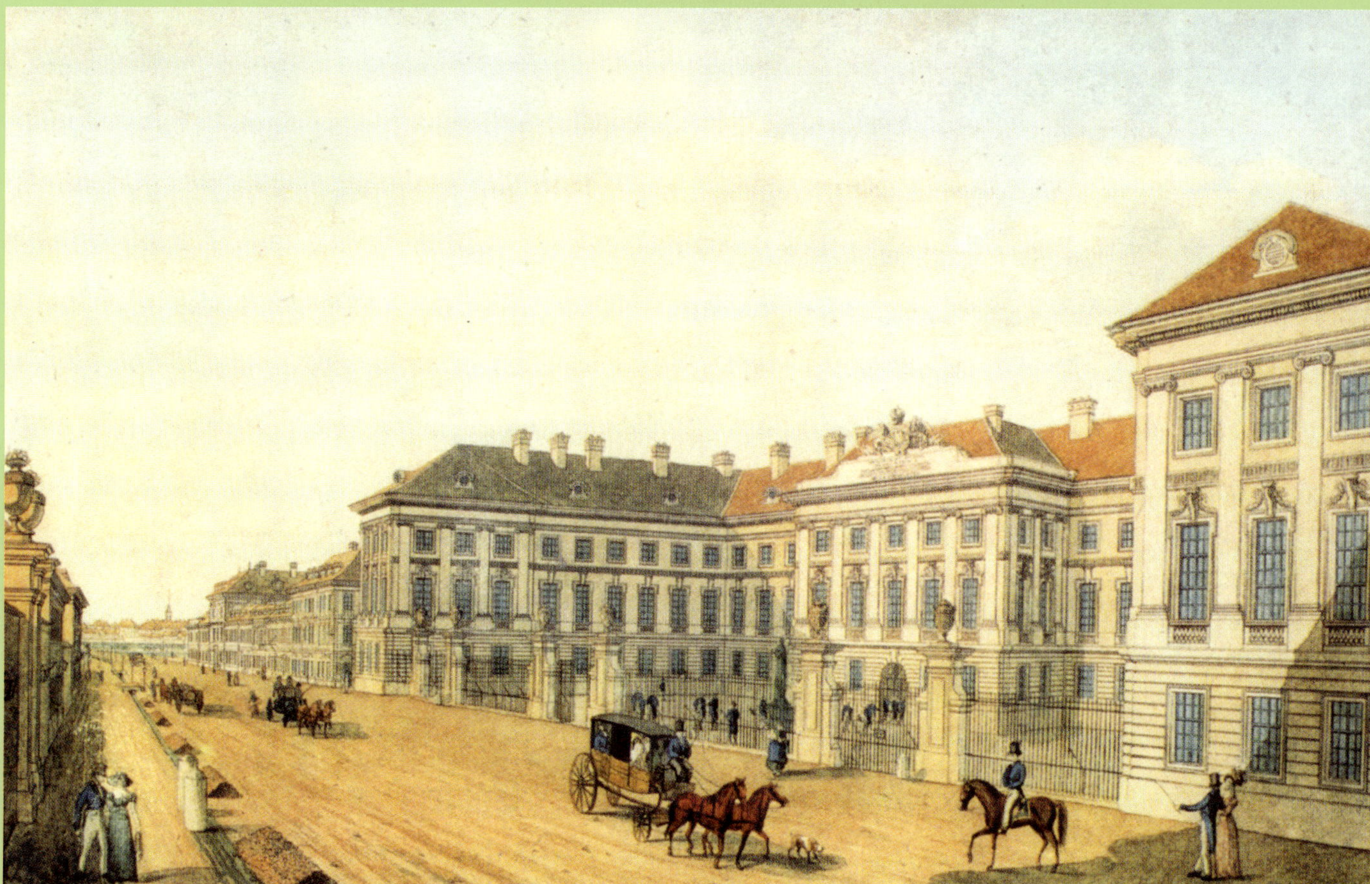

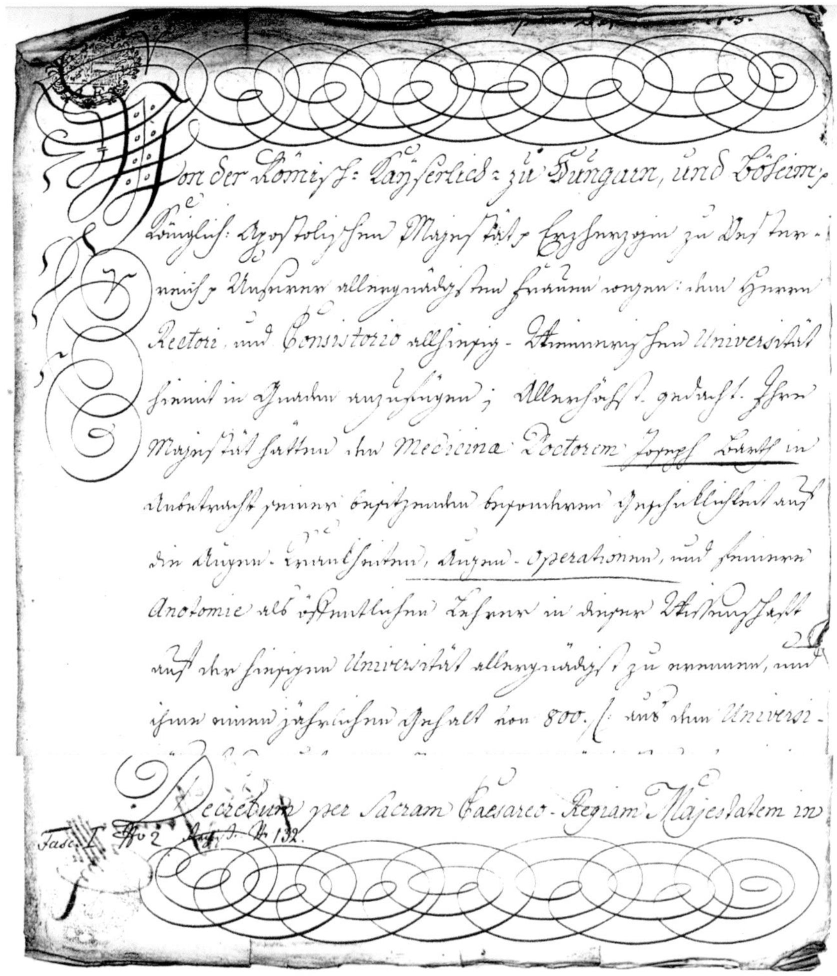

Fig. 3 a, b
Appointment of Joseph Barth (a) German (b) Latin

(a) translated from the German (abbreviated, photomontage): "From the Roman-Imperial, in Hungary and Bohemia Royal, Apostolic Majesty, Archduchess of Austria, our most gracious Lady … (Maria Theresa) … Her Majesty appointed Medicinae Doctorem Joseph Barth on account of his skill in eye diseases and eye surgery as public teacher in the local university…"continued at the bottom of page and overleaf: "Decretum per Sacram Caesareo-Regiam Majestatem in Consilio Cancellariae Bohemio-Austriaco Aulicae Viennae, Die 23tia Mensis Octobris Anno Domini 1773tio

(b)please read underlined text: …"Barth Professor Anatomiae et oculorum morborum ac Consiliarius declaratur", this translates into.
Barth was declared Professor of anatomy and of eye diseases.

(b) This is proof that the German wording of public teacher ("öffentlicher Lehrer") indicated the position of "Professor" at the University of Vienna (Acta Facultatis 1774)

Res inclytæ Facultatis

Revisio Rationum Facultatis.

Censor Rationum Facultatis et Societatis.

Crantz Professuram resignat.
Collin in illam transfertur.
Barth Professor Anatomiæ et oculorum morborum ac Consi-
liarius declaratur.
Heidele extraordinarius Lec-
tor Chirurgiæ et artis obste-
triciæ denominatur.
Decani electio quomodo in-
stituenda.

Institutum Facultatis me-
dicæ ab Augma confirmatum.

ad: 22. Ma

Rationes
binis Dnis
approbato
ad cassam
Post morten
ut Senior c
loco etiam
qui nunc c
re diversi
Congregat
Augma 1=
„care conc
Collin tran
„sorem Ana
Ejusque Co
Heidele en
„tis obstetr
fuit, quod
„ten perma
plurima v
non ampli
quo debitus
„datas et po
non integre
intimare, e
que proroga
5= tandem
medicæ Fa
mandato, u

Fig. 4

Frontispiece of vol 1 part 1 of Ophthalmologische Bibliothek, Braunschweig 1802

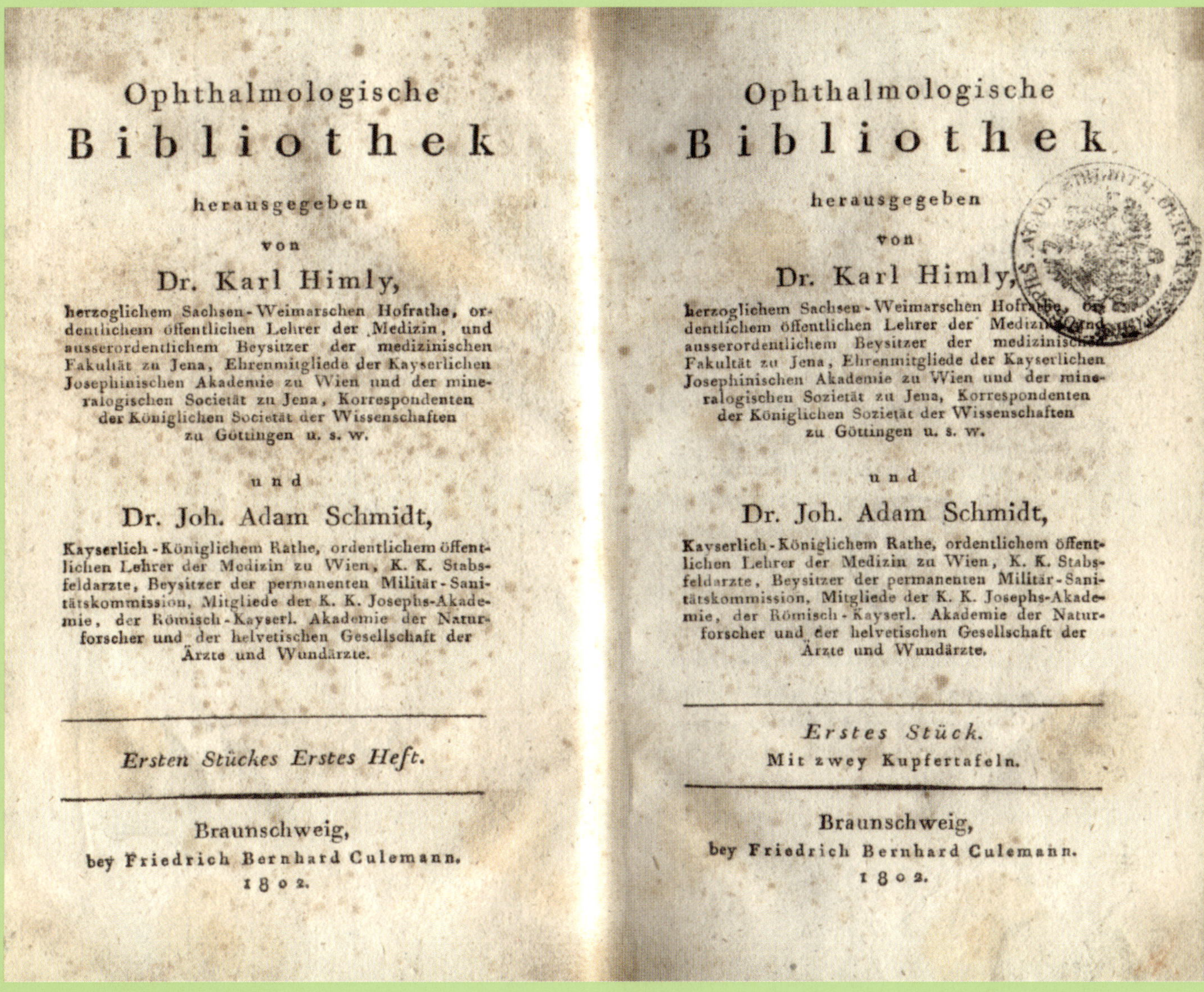

Ophthalmologische

Bibliothek

herausgegeben

von

Dr. Karl Himly,

herzoglichem Sachsen-Weimarschen Hofrathe, ordentlichem öffentlichen Lehrer der Medizin, und ausserordentlichem Beysitzer der medizinischen Fakultät zu Jena, Ehrenmitgliede der Kayserlichen Josephinischen Akademie zu Wien und der mineralogischen Societät zu Jena, Korrespondenten der Königlichen Societät der Wissenschaften zu Göttingen u. s. w.

und

Dr. Joh. Adam Schmidt,

Kayserlich-Königlichem Rathe, ordentlichem öffentlichen Lehrer der Medizin zu Wien, K. K. Stabsfeldarzte, Beysitzer der permanenten Militär-Sanitätskommission, Mitgliede der K. K. Josephs-Akademie, der Römisch-Kayserl. Akademie der Naturforscher und der helvetischen Gesellschaft der Ärzte und Wundärzte.

Ersten Stückes Erstes Heft.

Braunschweig,

bey Friedrich Bernhard Culemann.

1802.

Ophthalmologische

Bibliothek

herausgegeben

von

Dr. Karl Himly,

herzoglichem Sachsen-Weimarschen Hofrathe, ordentlichem öffentlichen Lehrer der Medizin, und ausserordentlichem Beysitzer der medizinischen Fakultät zu Jena, Ehrenmitgliede der Kayserlichen Josephinischen Akademie zu Wien und der mineralogischen Sozietät zu Jena, Korrespondenten der Königlichen Sozietät der Wissenschaften zu Göttingen u. s. w.

und

Dr. Joh. Adam Schmidt,

Kayserlich-Königlichem Rathe, ordentlichem öffentlichen Lehrer der Medizin zu Wien, K. K. Stabsfeldarzte, Beysitzer der permanenten Militär-Sanitätskommission, Mitgliede der K. K. Josephs-Akademie, der Römisch-Kayserl. Akademie der Naturforscher und der helvetischen Gesellschaft der Ärzte und Wundärzte.

Erstes Stück.

Mit zwey Kupfertafeln.

Braunschweig,

bey Friedrich Bernhard Culemann.

1802.

The Water–colours and Drawings from 1782 on, Clinical and Histopathologic: an individual evaluation by ophthalmologists

Edward Jaeger, Robert Nussenblatt, Günther Grabner, Hans Slezak and Anselm Kampik

Description of pictures by Edward Jaeger, ophthalmologist

Fig. 5
Painted by Dr. Georg Joseph Beer in 1786, for Dr. Joseph Barth (1745-1818), the first professor also for eye surgery and eye diseases, in Vienna.

On this painting Beer signed for the first time "Jos. Beer M.Dr."
Marked exophthalmos of the left eye is shown in this painting of a 30-40 year old male. The proptosis appears solid and more prominent superiorly pushing the eye downward. The normal ocular structures are not recognizable. The patient does not appear otherwise debilitated.

The picture is consistent with an orbital tumor although an intraocular lesion cannot be totally discounted. There are a wide variety of tumor possibilities which include lymphoma/leukemia, optic nerve glioma, Ewings sarcoma, orbital hemangioma and neurofibroma. The patient's apparent age would mitigate against a rhabdomyosarcoma, which occurs in children. However, a rhabdomyosarcoma is flesh colored and most commonly occurs in the superior orbit. While the proptosis appears solid, a parasitic orbital cyst cannot entirely be ruled out on the basis of the drawing.

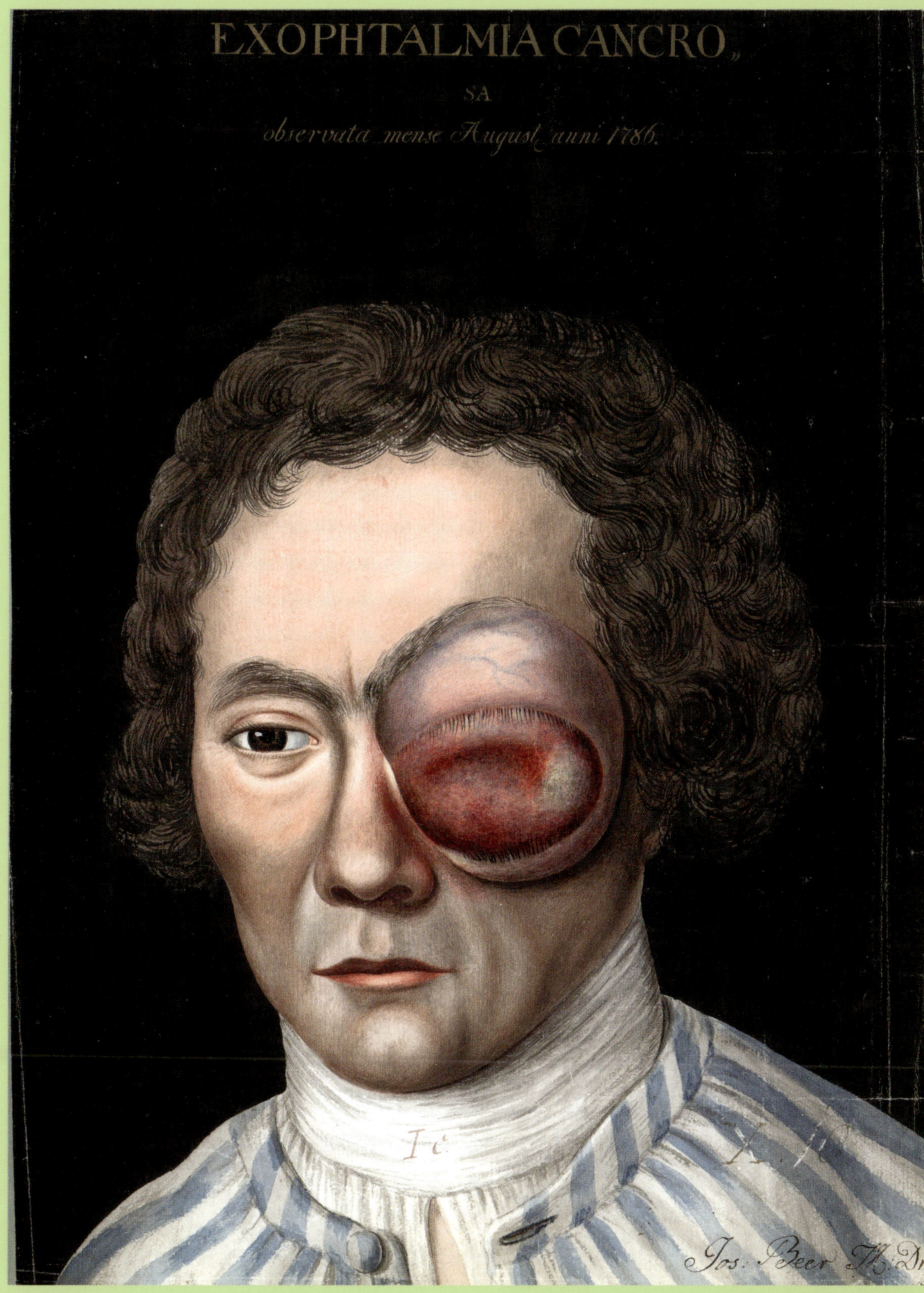
EXOPHTALMIA CANCRO,
SA
observata mense August anni 1786.
Jos: Beer M: Dr

Fig. 6
Painted by Dr. Georg Joseph Beer, 1816

This drawing shows an inflamed upper lid and a gross reddish protuberance which has replaced the normal ocular structure. The exophthalmos in this lady is consistent with orbital infiltration by the canine tapeworm, Echinococcus granulosus. This parasite produces characteristic tissue cysts throughout the body. This condition also is referred to as hydatid disease. The eye is not recognizable as such in this drawing.

The dog is the definitive host for the Echinococcus organism with sheep, cattle and pigs serving as intermediate host. Ingested eggs are hatched in the human intestine and the larvae travel via the blood stream to various organs where they form hydatid cysts. Ocular involvement may be orbital or intraocular.

Exophtalmus hydatoideus. No. $\frac{337}{68}$. A $\frac{1815}{1816}$

8. ~~VIII~~

II b.

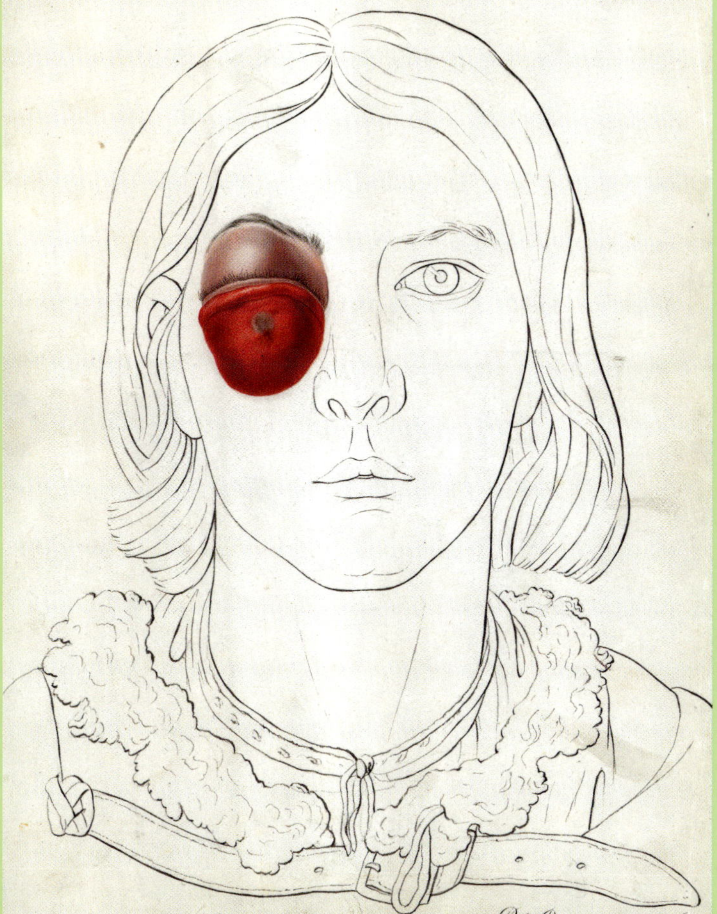

Prof. Beer a. n. pinx. 1816.

Fig. 7
Painted likely by Dr. Georg Joseph Beer

The drawing is a lateral view of a lady with extensive chemosis involving the right ocular and orbital areas. The edema is contained within the orbital septum area. The upper eyelid appears to be intact but the lower lid is not recognizable. The status of the globe cannot be determined. The irregular circle toward the nose most likely represents the cornea.

This picture could result from an intraocular or orbital tumor, although trauma and orbital cellulitis cannot be ruled out.

The picture seems to depict the same patient as in the foregoing image, perhaps at a later stage.

b. ix.

IIc.

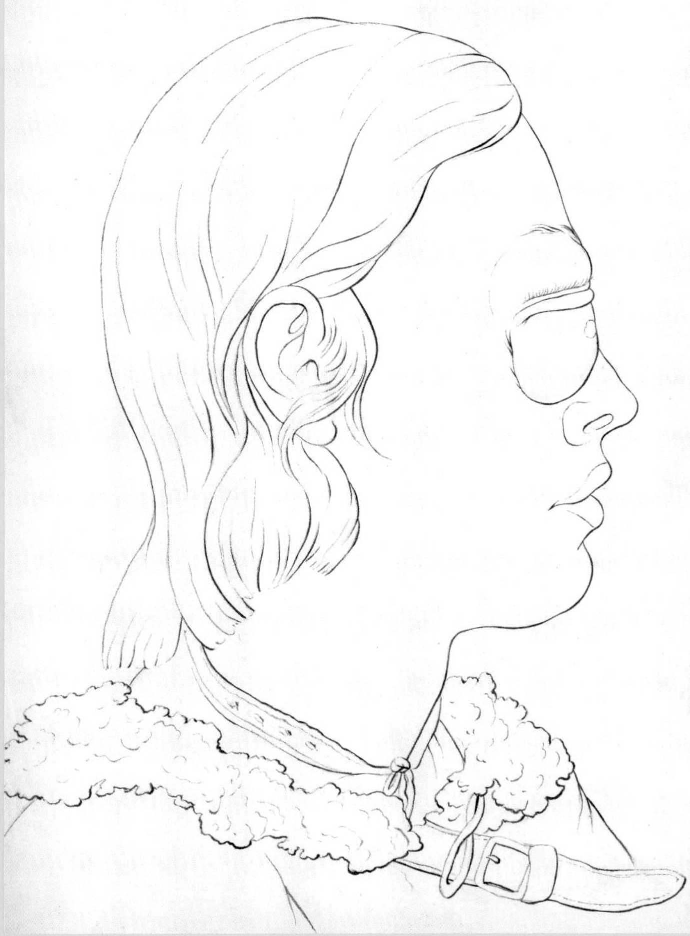

Fig. 8
By Jos. Zehner 1830/1831

A young female is shown with a prominent protuberance, staphyloma, of the left eye. The anterior surface of the staphyloma is pigmented and finely nodular, replacing the normal architecture of the anterior segment. A diffuse, bluish-black pigmentation is present for 8–10 millimeters posterior to the limbus, the thinnest portion of the sclera. Some pigment also is seen in the mid-portion of the left lower lid. These ocular findings are accentuated in the lateral view.

The staphyloma could represent the forward extension of an anterior segment melanoma. A speculative but interesting etiology is that of ocular melanocytosis or Nevus of Ota syndrome. There is an increased incidence of malignant melanoma in this condition. Another possibility is a traumatic intra-uterine or birth injury causing a ruptured globe.

In such cases, the iris sometimes may seal the hole. However, glaucoma frequently develops, creating the staphyloma.

N° VII.

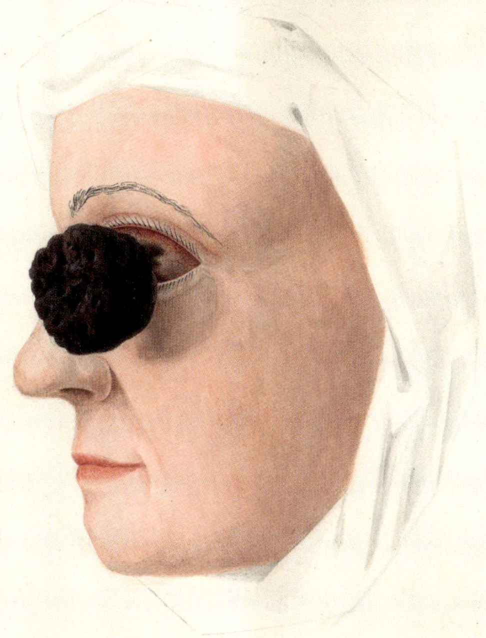

Melanosis bulbi oculi.
Protocollirt im Schuljahr $18\frac{30}{31}$ N° 104.

Jos. Zehner.

Fig. 9

This drawing of an adult woman shows symmetric narrowing of the palpebral fissures, drooping of the eyelids and absence of the normal horizontal upper eyelid fold. Epicanthal folds extend laterally, both inferiorly and superiorly, different from the more common ethnically related epicanthal folds. There appears to be a wider than normal distance between the medial canthi.

This picture is consistent with a congenital defect now termed Blepharophimosis, Epicanthus Inversus and Ptosis Syndrome*. However, the usually flat nose bridge is not present. Recent genetic studies have indicated an associated chromosomal abnormality. The term blepharophimosis is frequently used to describe this picture and it may be associated with other syndromes having multiple and varied systemic manifestations.

* Brooks BP, Traboulsi EI. Congenital Malformations of the Eye in Tasman W. Jaeger EA (eds): Foundations of Clinical Ophthalmology. Lippincott, Williams and Wilkins, Philadelphia 2000: volume I, Ch 40: 15-16

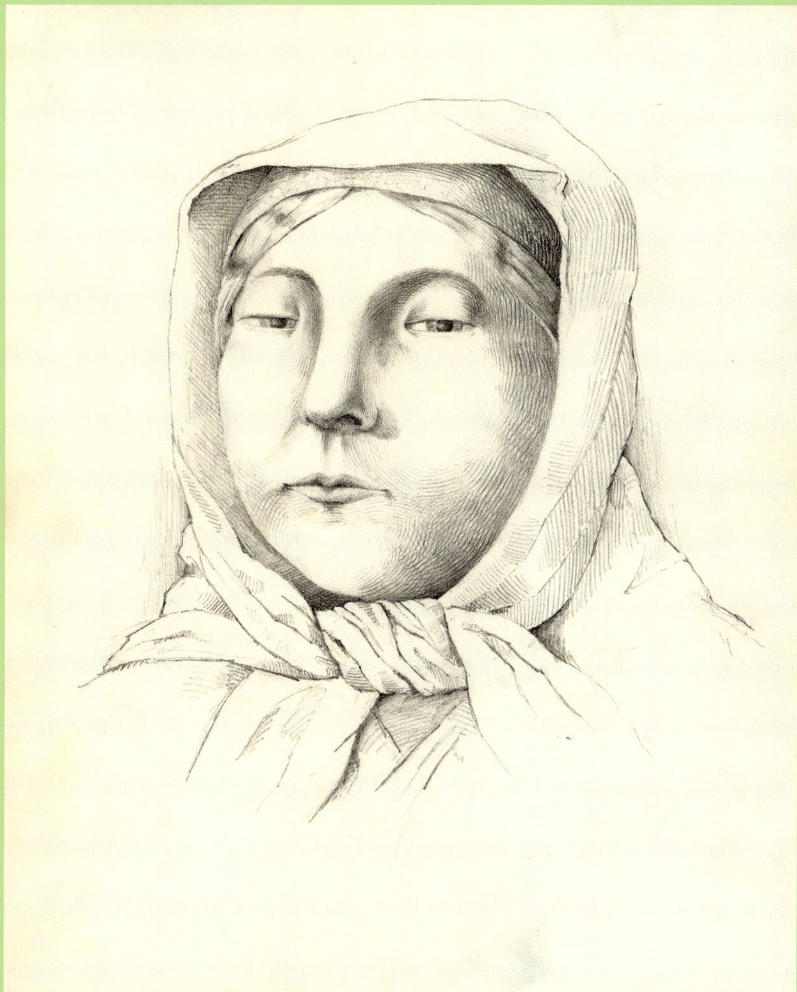

Fig. 10
By the brush of Dr. Carl von Rzehaczek, 1844, Ferdinand Hebra's pal and painter, later professor of surgery in Graz

An irregular, nodular melanotic mass fills the anterior segment of the left eye resulting in a solid appearing anterior staphyloma in this patient. The normal structures are not visible and the eye appears inflamed.

This picture would be consistent with a melanoma of the iris or anterior ciliary body. This drawing is very similar to one done by Professor Joseph Beer that also appears in this collection.

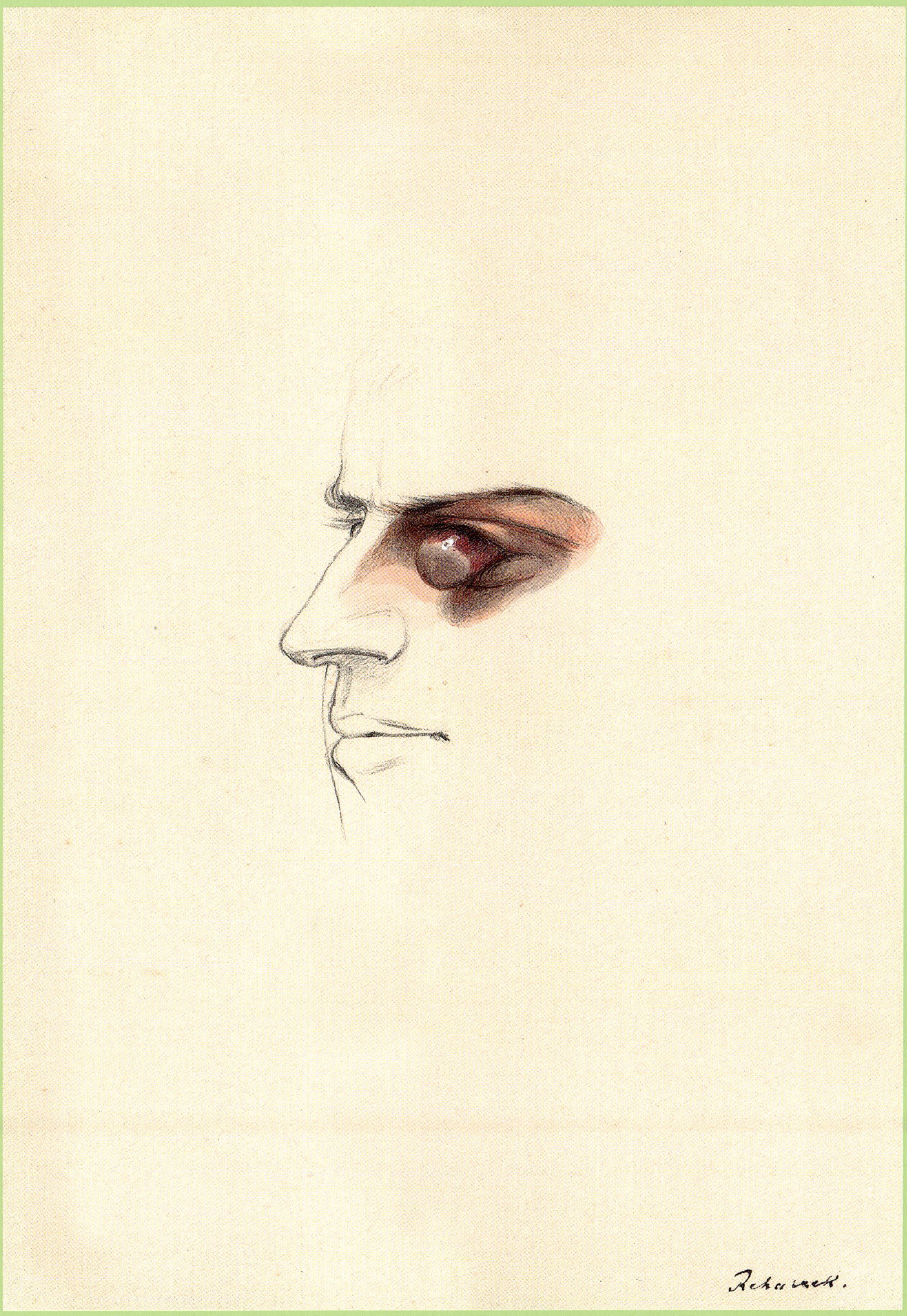

Fig. 12
A fairly dense, diffuse opacification of the lens is recorded in this painting. A small, less opaque zone is noted inferiorly. The lens opacity represents a moderate degree of nuclear sclerosis. The globe itself appears larger than normal, perhaps indicating a myopic eye. Another possibility is a superiorly dislocated lens such as might occur with Marfan syndrome.

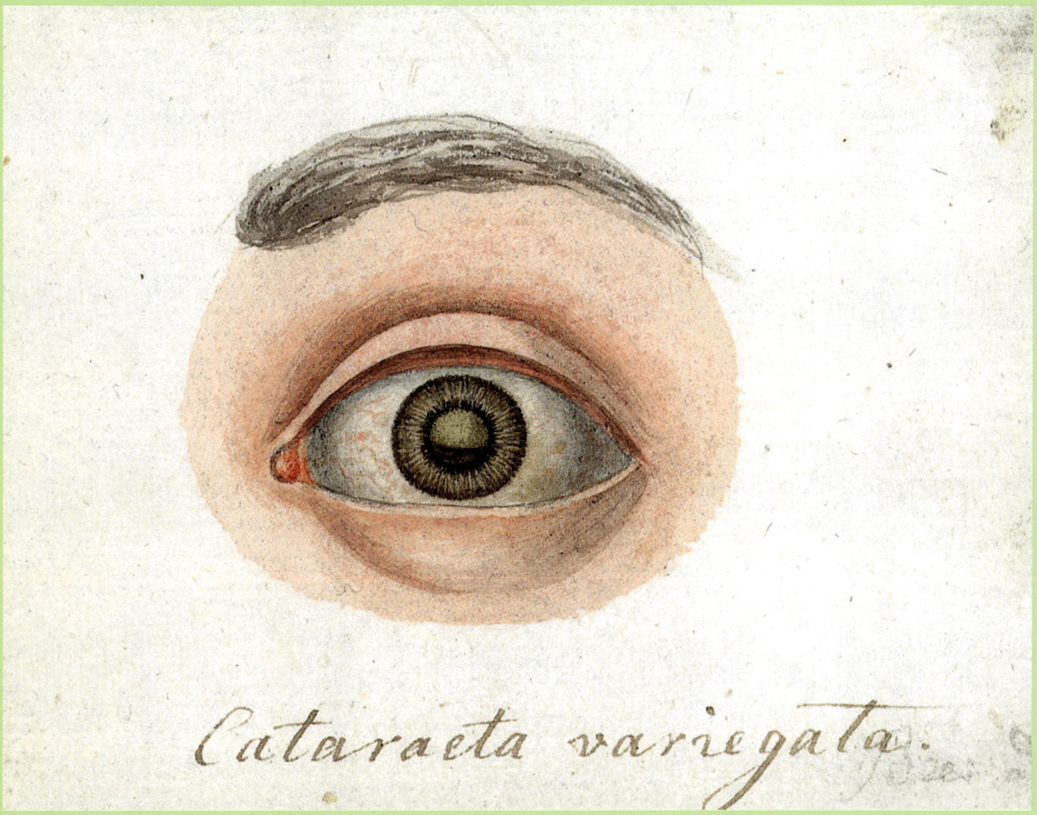
Cataracta variegata.

Fig.13
By Dr. Georg Joseph Beer's brush 1791

This painting shows differences in coloration of the irides in the eyes of a young patient. The iris of the right eye is brown and the left blue, indicating less melanotic pigment in the left eye. The right eye appears esotropic. Radial striations are noted in the iris of both eyes. The eyes are otherwise unremarkable except for a haze in the lens of the left eye in the pupillary area.

Heterochromia iridum has a wide spectrum of etiologies. The condition may be present at birth and a hereditary association has been documented. A variety of disease processes may result in acquired heterochromia. One of the most common is Fuch's heterochromic iridocyclitis in which a chronic anterior uveitis results in stromal atrophy of the ipsilateral iris and consequently, a lighter color. Glaucoma and cataract formation as may be the case in this patient are frequent complications. In cases in which the lighter eye is the normal, the darker iris could represent a melanoma.

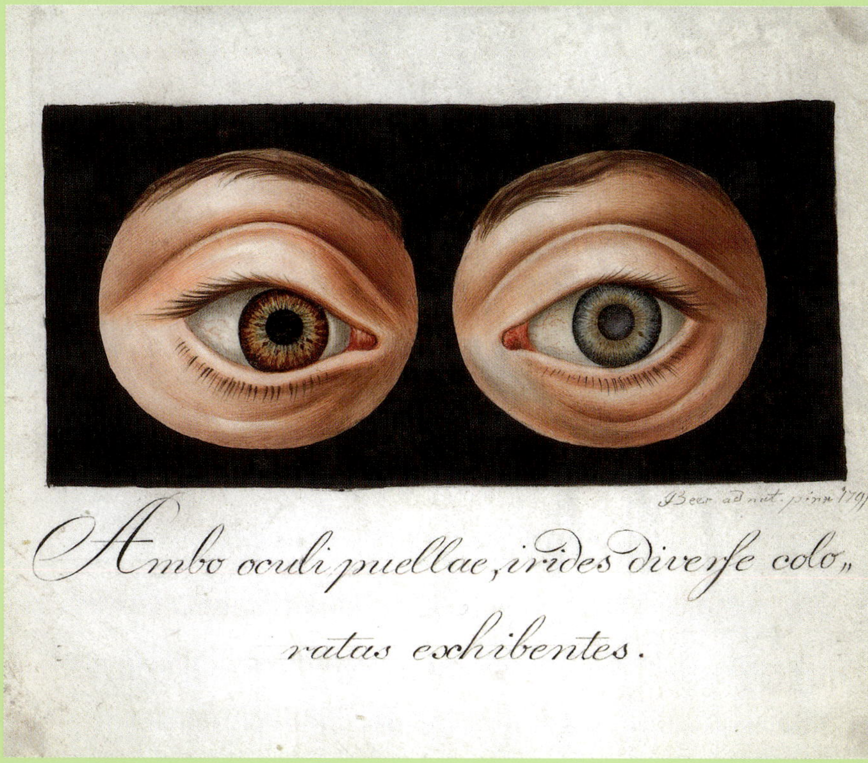
J Beer ad nat. pinx 1797
Ambo oculi puellae, irides diverſe colo„
ratas exhibentes.

Fig. 14
By Dr. Georg Joseph Beer 1814

The anterior surface of the cornea has a diffuse, dark coloration with nodular grape-like staphyloma in the inferior temporal quadrant. The eye is grossly congested and the normal anterior segment architecture is not visible.

This most likely represents the anterior extension of a malignant melanoma of the iris or anterior ciliary body. The painting is remarkably similar to another illustration in this series painted by Dr. Carl von Rzehaczek.

Staphyloma racemosum.

ad No. $\frac{105}{28}$ A $\frac{1813}{14}$. Intr.

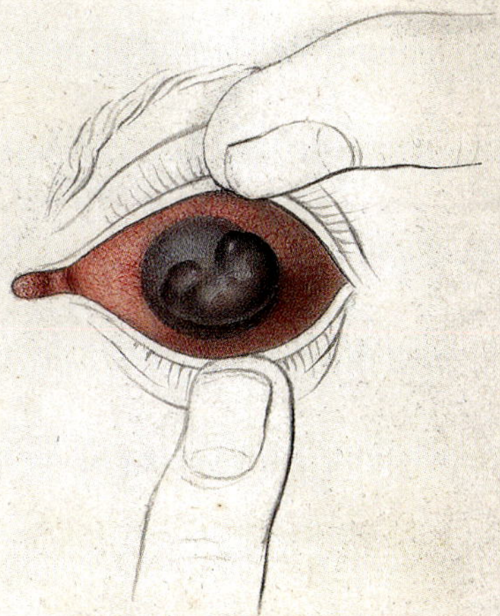

Prof. Beer ad nat. p.
1814.

Fig. 16
Most likely by Dr. Georg Joseph Beer 1817/1818

A wedge-shaped, thick fleshy growth extends from the superior fornix to the inferior margin of the cornea. An adhesion to the cornea is present at the apex of this membrane. The eye appears injected and there is dilation of the perilimbal vessels, indicative of an active inflammatory process.

This growth is not a true pterygium because of its vertical orientation and is probably inflammatory in etiology. A pterygium, in our present day terminology, is a horizontal extension of vascularized tissue onto the cornea, usually from the nasal limbus and within the exposed palpebral fissure area. Solar radiation is felt to be the etiologic stimulus for such a growth.

It would be reasonable to assume that a corneal ulcer had been present in this patient with long standing inflammation resulting in the overgrowth of this fibrovascular membrane. The most likely diagnosis is phlyctenulosis keratitis associated with a tubercular infection. However, other granulomatous diseases such as syphilis and sarcoidosis, as well as invasion of the cornea by other bacterial or viral organisms could conceivably result in this picture.

Pterygium sarcomatosum.

Ad № $\frac{769}{152}$ p. a. $\frac{1817}{1818}$.

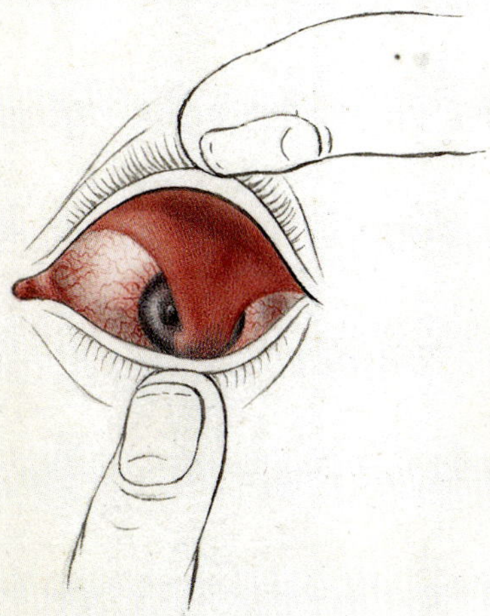

Fig. 17
By Dr. Carl Heitzmann (1836–1896) 1864, dermatologist and pathologist, Hebra's third painter, later founding member of the American Dermatological Association, 1876, elder brother of Dr. Julius Heitzmann, who continued painting in Vienna for the rest of the century

Upper Right: The pupil in this patient is constricted with iris pigment deposition on the lens surface and an opaque coloration to the anterior lens surface. A small, soft, whitish tuft (floccule) is seen at the inferior pupil margin. Upper Left: The pupil has been dilated and pigment deposition along with posterior synechia is apparent. Lower Left: Some of the synechiae have been broken by dilation. Additional floccules are noted. Lower Right: Inflammatory membranes are present on the anterior surface of the iris and considerable debris has accumulated on the anterior lens surface. Opacification of the anterior lens surface is apparent and neovascularization is noted on the anterior surface of the iris and lens.

These four paintings illustrate the inflammatory involvement of the anterior segment of the eye in a patient with chronic anterior uveitis. The synechia formation, the inflammatory membranes, lens opacification with new vessel formation and increasing floccule formation attest to the chronicity of the inflammatory process.

The anterior segment is in sharp focus mitigating against a granulomatous process in which the cornea would be clouded by mutton-fat keratoprecipitates.

The small white floccules most likely are inflammatory residues. They are not entirely characteristic of Koeppe or Busacca nodules. Koeppe nodules cling to the anterior iris surface and Busacca nodules usually are intrastromal near the pupillary margin. Both are somewhat darker and associated with a granulomatous process. Berliner preferred to call these formations efflorescences because of their histologic composition, which varied from coagulated fibrin, sometimes with cells, to more solid structure with granulomatous cells and caseation.

Many practitioners of the day felt these were associated with syphilis or tuberculosis.

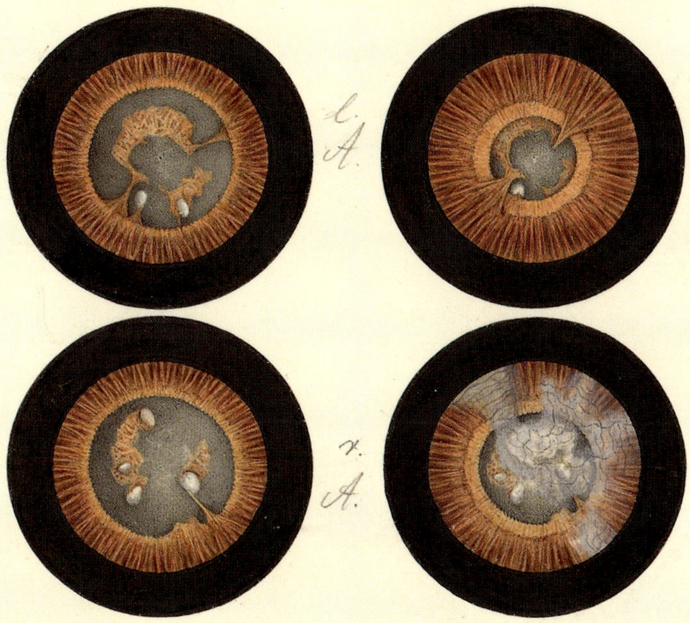

Dr Heitzmann fec.

Fig. 18
By Dr. Carl Heitzmann 1865

This painting shows dramatic new vessel formation over the surface of the cornea with a concentration in the inferior nasal quadrant. The iris is not distorted and the neovascularization appears limited to the external surface of the eye. The perilimbal vessels are dilated and the pupil miotic indicating an accompanying anterior uveitis. No focal corneal scarring or limbal nodules are seen.

The possible etiologic stimuli for this vascularization are varied and multiple. Untreated recurrent herpes simplex keratitis is one of the more common causes of corneal neovascularization. Although the vascularization appears mostly superficial, interstitial keritites associated with congenital syphilis, is another possibility. Chronic allergic keratoconjunctivitis also may result in such a picture. The absence of limbal phlyctenules would appear to rule out tuberculosis as a causative agent. However, in all of these possible etiologies, more corneal involvement than is shown would have been anticipated.

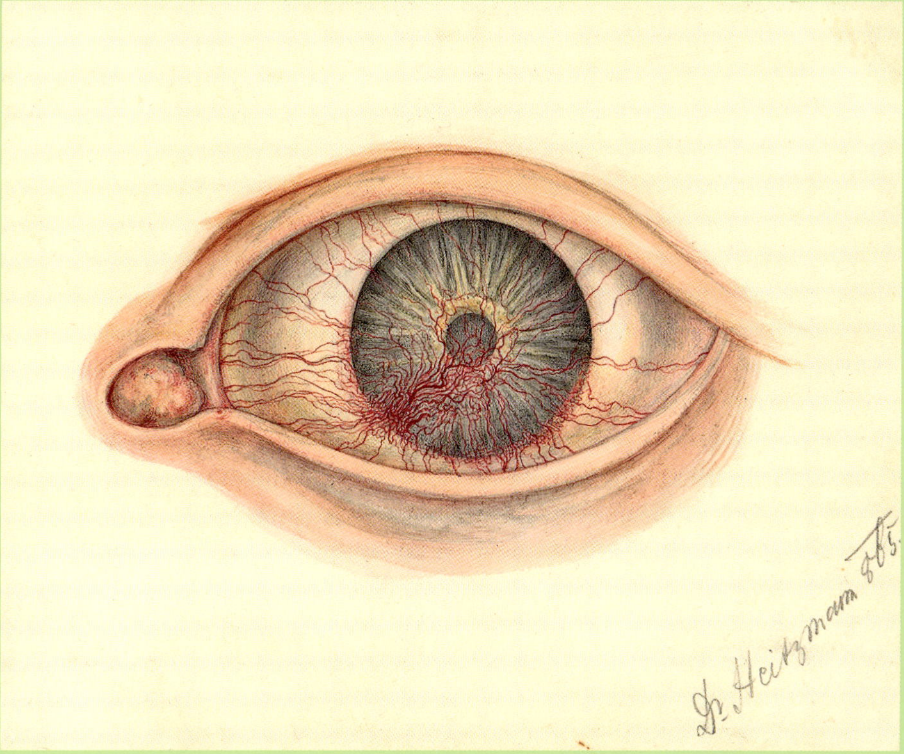
Dr. Heitzmann 885.

Fig. 20
Obviously by Dr. Carl Heitzmann

This painting is likely a follow-up of the previous patient in the above illustration. The tumor mass now has completely destroyed the normal architecture of the left eye, which has been displaced laterally. The tumor surface has become irregular, filling the orbit and is protruding anteriorly. The inferior lid margin is irregular, suggesting possible necrosis. The upper lid is entropic.

The most likely diagnosis in this young lady appears to be that of a retinoblastoma but other intraocular conditions such as parasitic cysts and the orbital extension of a malignant melanoma cannot be ruled out.

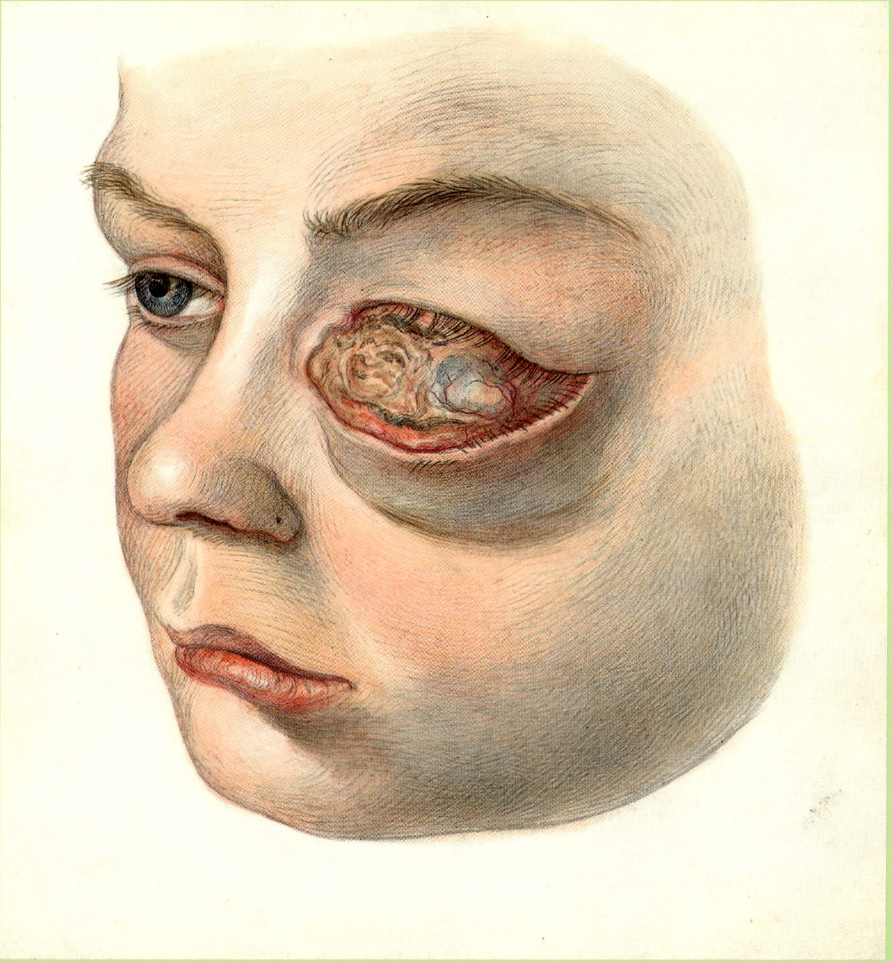

Fig. 21
By Dr. Eduard Jaeger 1866

This painting illustrates subretinal cysticercosis, which was common in Germany and Austria in the 18th and 19th centuries. There is pallor, edema and folds of the inferior retina. Two darker, circular areas probably representing anterior retinal holes are visible. The scolex of the worm is visible centrally beneath the retinal surface. The inferior disc margin is edematous.

Cysticercus is the larval form of Taenia solium, a tapeworm. After humans ingest eggs, the larvae penetrate the intestinal wall and are carried via the blood stream throughout the body, including all parts of the eye. Professor Jaeger described the undulating movements of the parasite seen through the retina.

This drawing is very similar to one that appears in Jaeger's Atlas of Diseases of the Ocular Fundus (1869 edition). This collection of drawings was sold to William Fisher Norris, M.D. for the sum of $ 2400. Dr. Norris had been a student under Professor Eduard Jaeger in 1865 at the Vienna Department. He subsequently became Professor of Ophthalmology at the University of Pennsylvania in Philadelphia, USA. Upon his death, the collection was bequeathed to the College of Physicians of Philadelphia. Daniel M. Albert, M.D. combined the illustrations into an atlas with English subtitles and descriptions. This book presently resides in the historical section of the College library.

Albert DM: Jaeger's Atlas of Diseases of the Ocular Fundus (1869 English edition). Saunders, Philadelphia, 1972.

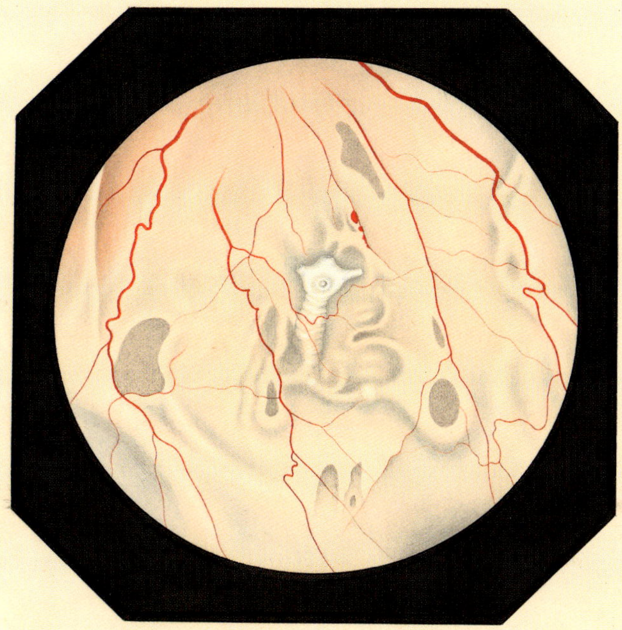

Dr. Jaeger jun. ad natur. del. 21/3 66.

Fig. 22
This fundus painting demonstrates the typical crescent shaped area of atrophy of the retinal pigment epithelium (RPE) and thinning of the choroid temporal to the disc of a highly myopic eye. The disc appears to be normal. There are patchy areas of RPE atrophy and pigment clumping in the macular area. The foveal pigmentation could represent a Fuch's spot, which is a hyperplasia of the RPE often associated with a previous underlying choroidal neovascular net that has undergone spontaneous resolution. Central vision, most likely, is considerably reduced in this patient.

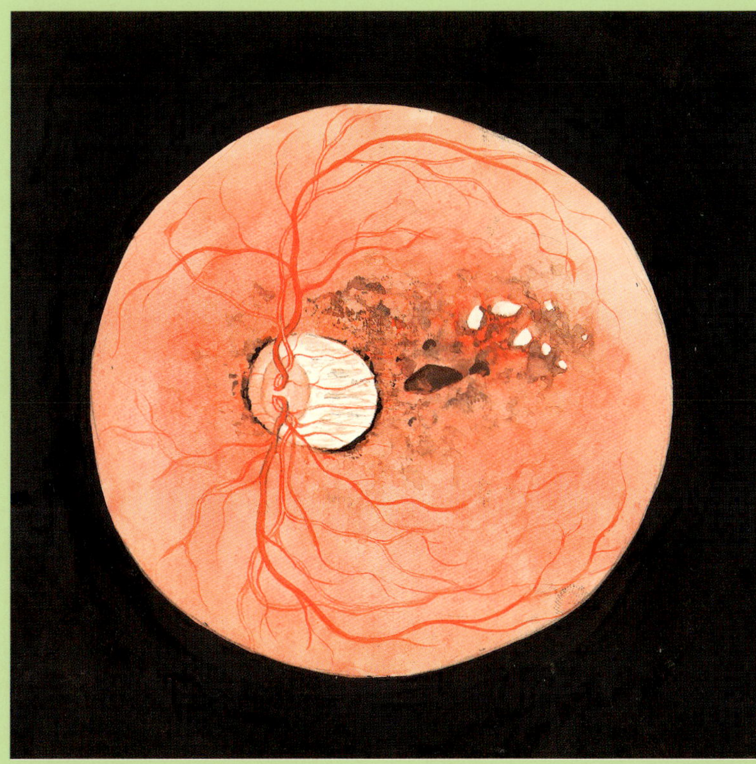

Description by Robert Nussenblatt, ophthalmologist

Fig. 23
By Jos. Zehner 1831/1832
This is a cross section of the skull showing a large mass in the vicinity of the left orbit. Only bony structures remain. Difficult to know if this originated from the eye or its adnexa.

116,

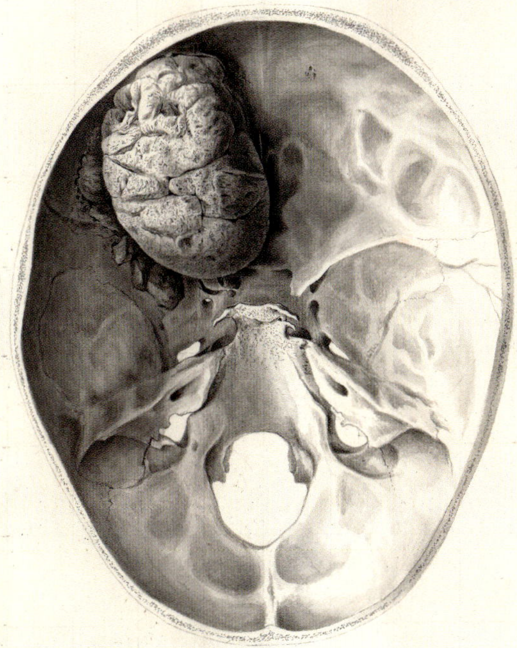

Exostosis orbitæ.

Protocollirt im Schuljahr $18\frac{31}{32}$ No 23.

Jos. Zehner

Fig. 24
By Dr. Carl von Rzehaczek, surgeon, Hebra's first painter 1844

The drawing shows a grossly abnormal left eye which protrudes beyond the lids. The cornea is not clear and could reflect the internal disorganization inside the eye. An enlargement of the globe could be due to long term high pressure inside in the eye or secondary to a tumor.

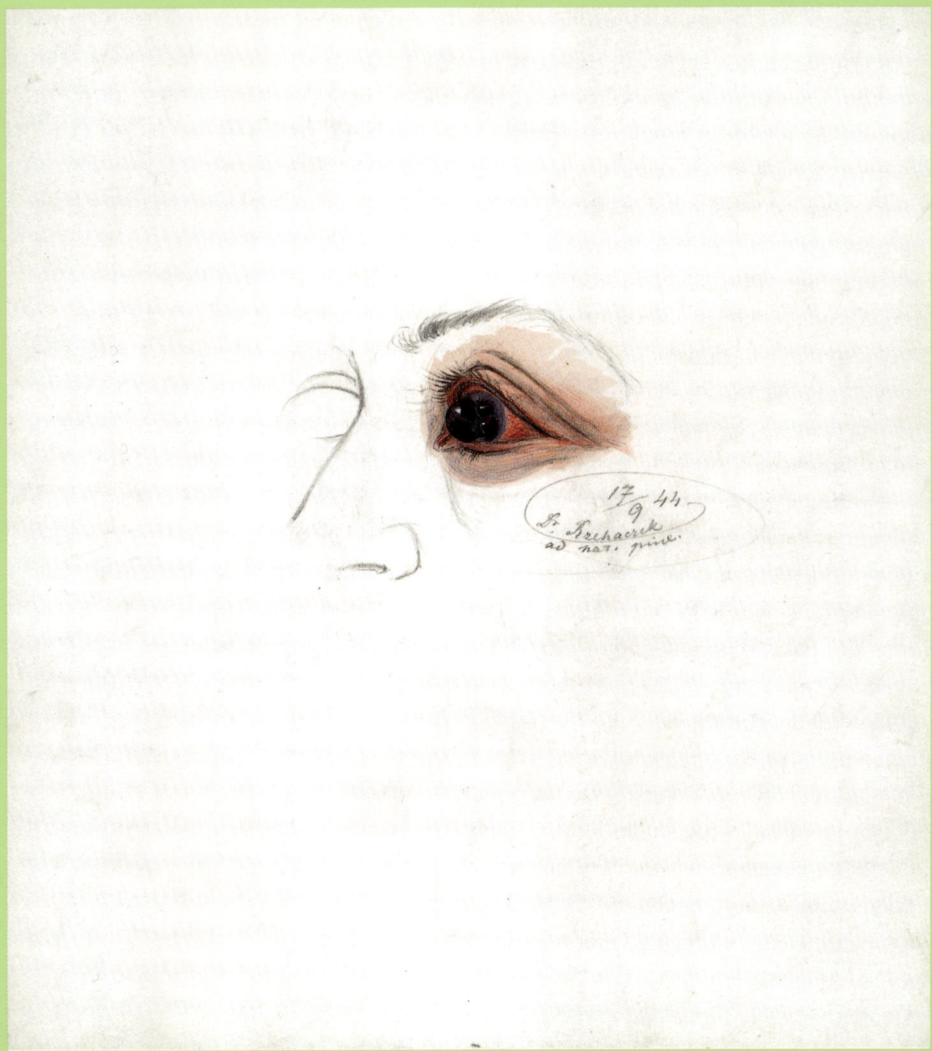
17/9 44
Dr. Krzhaczek
ad nat. pinx.

Figs. 26, 27
By Mayda, dedicated to Professor Anton von Rosas, Beer's successor in the chair up to 1855

It demonstrates an acute and chronic case of the same disease. This would be suggestive of follicular conjunctivitis. The acute form could be due to virus, such as adenovirus and in the chronic form this could be due to trachoma. The chronic form can then scar and in turn cause scarring of the cornea with blindness.

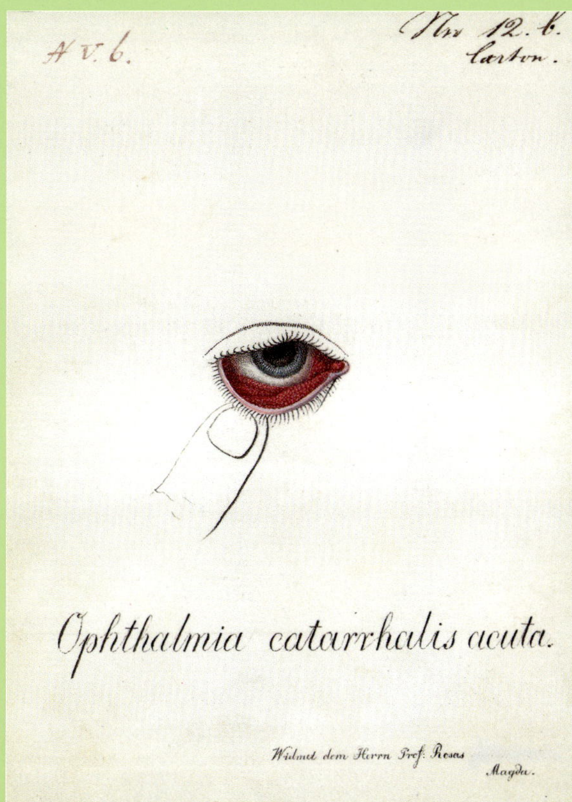
A V. b.
Nr 12. b.
carton.
Ophthalmia catarrhalis acuta.
Widmet dem Herrn Prof. Rosas
Magda.

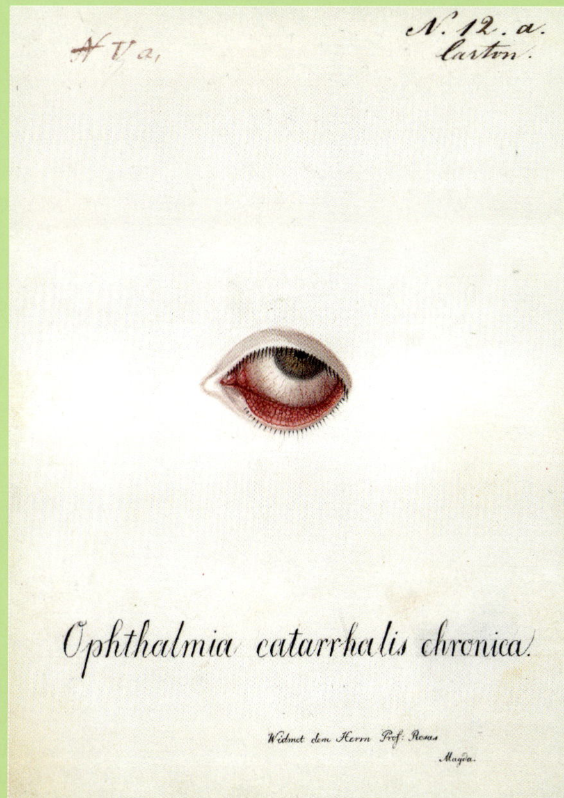
A V a.
N. 12. a.
carton.
Ophthalmia catarrhalis chronica.
Widmet dem Herrn Prof. Rosas
Magda.

Figs. 28, 29
By Dr. Georg Joseph Beer 1785

Appears to be the same person. These grotesque changes would suggest a slow growing lesion since a quick growing tumor would have killed the person before it got to this stage. The lesion may be due to neurofibromatosis causing this elephant like appearance. However, more recent evaluation would suggest that this presentation is more likely that of the Proteus Syndrome. The term Proteus Syndrome (named after the Greek god Proteus) was first used in 1983* to describe a disorder that is characterized by overgrowth of both bony and soft tissues. This can include hamartomatous lesions as well. In this picture the lesion involves the whole upper right front of the skull and has invaded the orbit. The contents of the orbit appear to be necrotic.

---

* Wiedemann HR, Burgio GR, Aldenhoff P et al.The Proteus syndrome: partial gigantism of the hands and/or feet, nevi, hemihypertrophy, subcutaneous tumors, macrocephaly, skull anomalies and possible accelerated growth and visceral affections. Eur J Pediatr 1983; 140:5-12

I a.

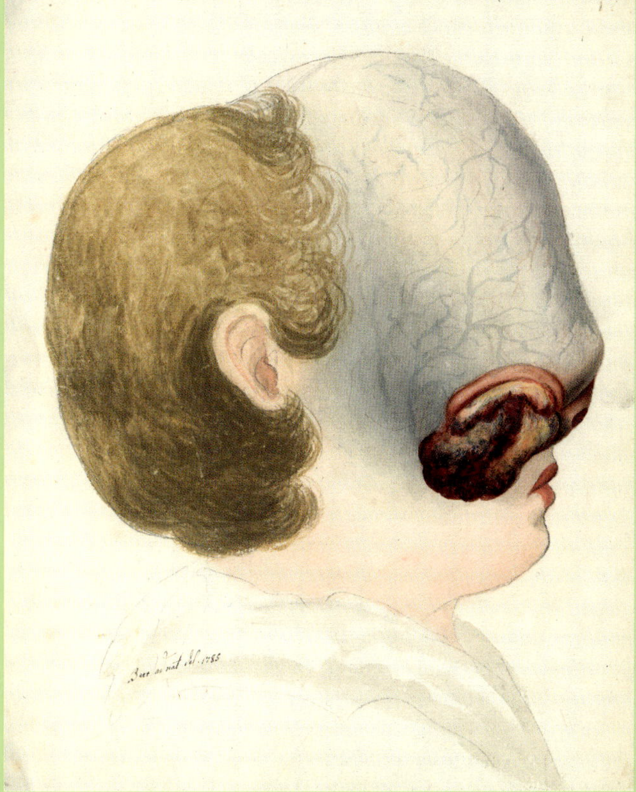

I b.

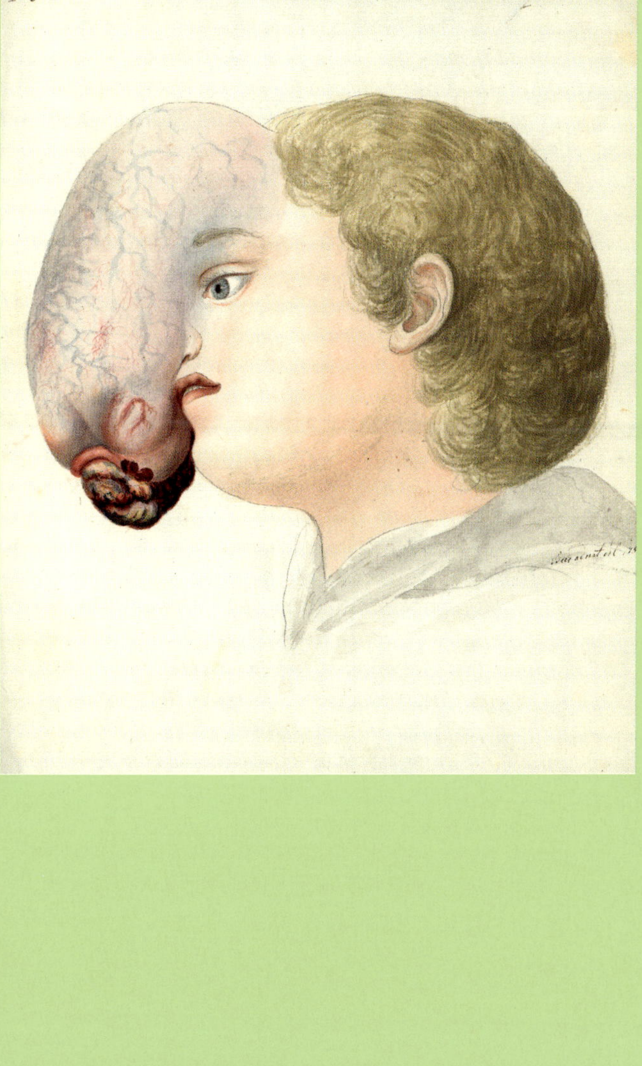

Fig. 30
By Dr. Carl Heitzmann 1863

The drawing states this is an example of anophthalmous or no eye. The lids are drawn up but there is a circular discoloration and swelling below the eyelids, perhaps in the lower portion of the eye extending under the skin. This could be hemorrhage but it is not clear what that would be from.

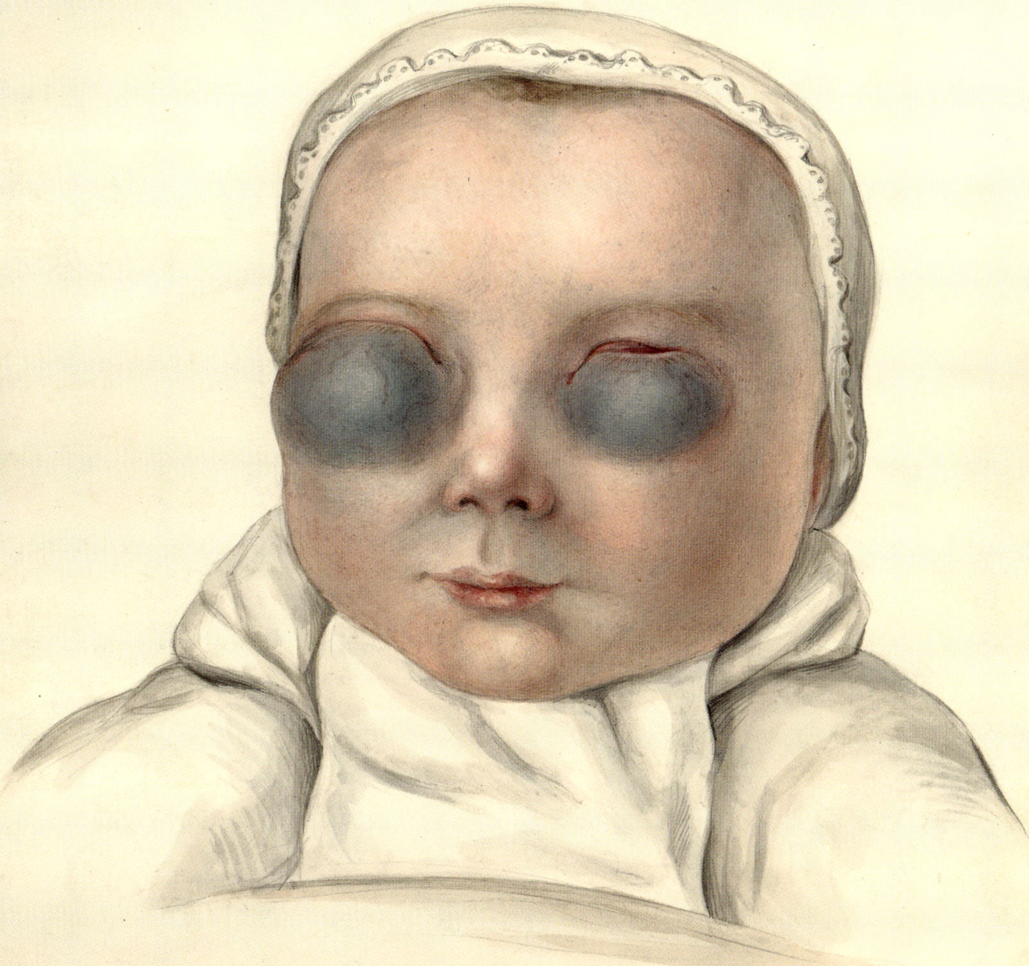

Schnobl Johann aus Preßburg
geb. 1862. Mutter desselben
mit microphth. oc. sin.

Anophthalmus.

Fig. 31
By Dr. Ed. Prochaska 1888

The drawing shows a right eye with someone keeping the lids open. The cornea is not clear and shows what could be a penetrating injury through the cornea. One can see a hole and white surrounding it, typical of a corneal injury. The eye is red and certainly painful. The structures of the anterior chamber of the eye are not distinct because of the injury which has almost certainly caused an hemorrhage and probably an infection.

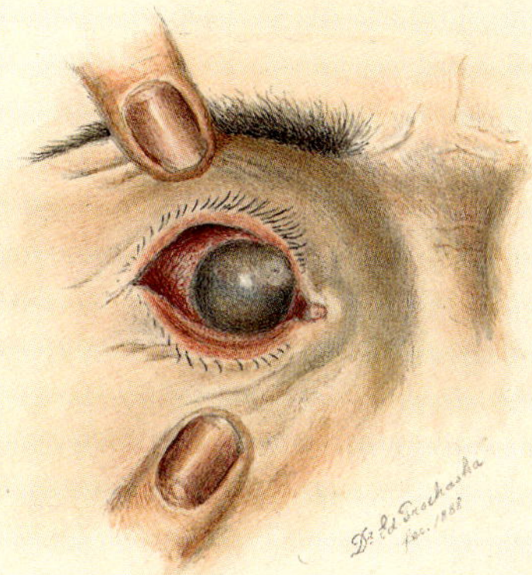
Dr. Ed. Prochaska

Fig. 32
By Dr. Carl von Rzehaczek 1843

This full face drawing shows that both eyes are affected. One possibility is trauma and an inflammatory response to both eyes, and the lesion below the left eye may speak to that. The lids are markedly distorted and either adherent to the globe or parts of the lid structure are missing leaving the nasal portion of the globe exposed. Another possibility is that of ocular pemphigoid, which would involve the mucosal membranes surrounding the globe. It would seem less likely because of the swollen lid on the left and the signs of a wound beneath that.

N. XVI

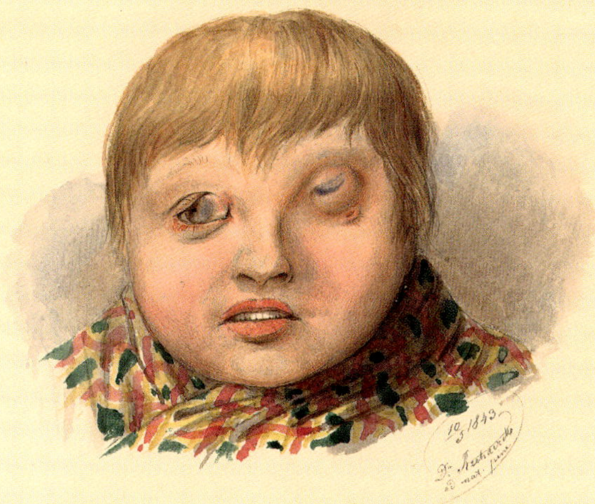

Fig. 33
By Jos. Zehner, 1830/1831

The drawing is labeled Melanosis bulbi oculi which indeed it is. This would appear to be melanoma that has extended from the ocular conjunctiva or began in the anterior segment of the eye and extended outward beyond the globe and involves the periocular structures as well. This would have a high risk of metastases to the liver.

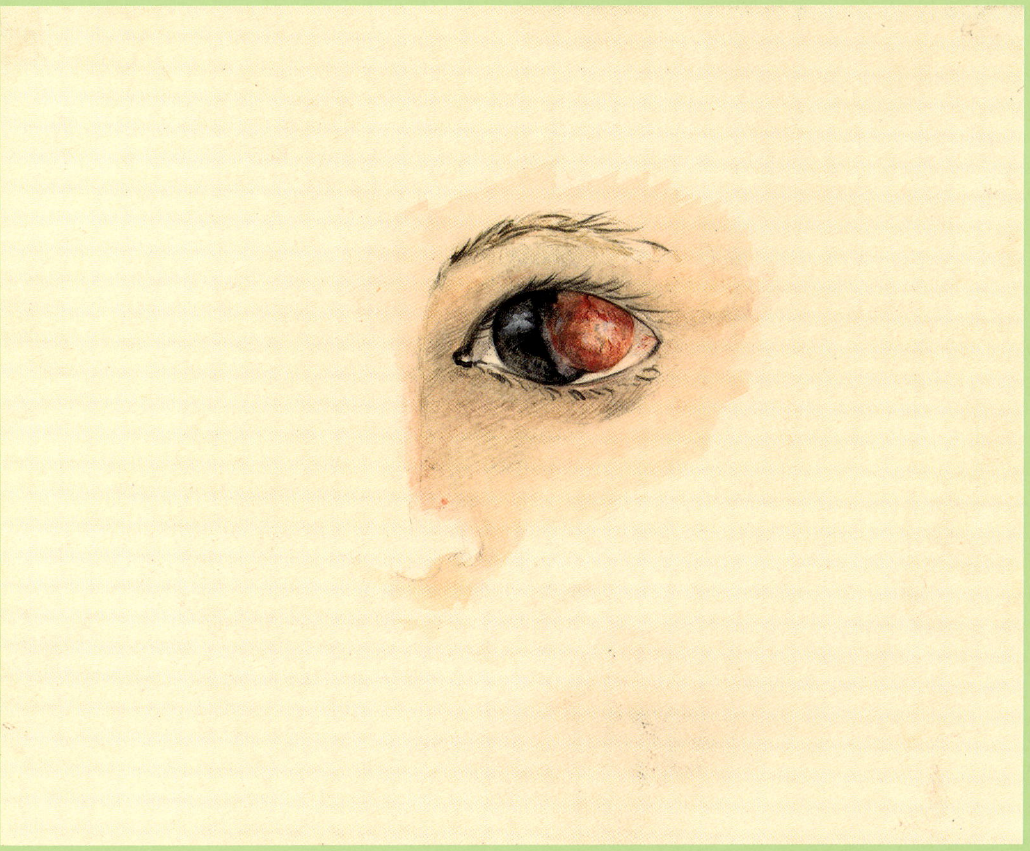

Fig. 34
By Dr. Carl Heitzmann 1867

This left eye is being propped open and probably is painful. The conjunctiva is inflamed. Centrally there is a large fleshy lesion sitting in the center of the cornea. Inflamed conjunctival tissue has come down from the superior aspect to join with the lesion centrally. This phenomenon is probably reflective of a chronic process suggestive a long standing irritation. It may have begun with an injury to the cornea with trauma or infection.

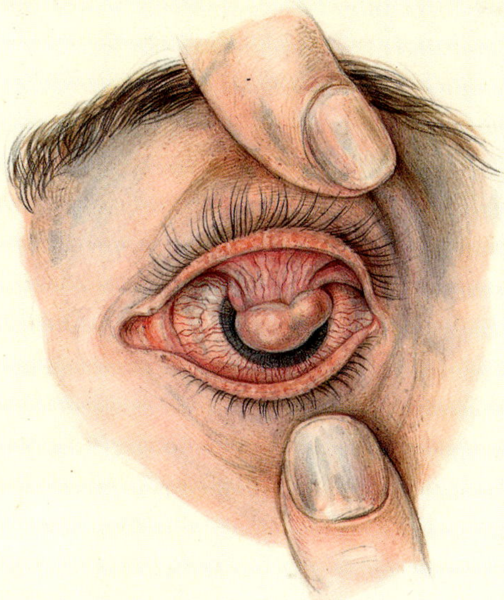

Grimm Julia 8t. Nov. 867.

Fig. 35

The iris architecture is distorted. This is a typical posterior synechia, an adhesion of the iris to the lens. The point of adhesion is evident on the drawing. This is typically seen as a result of an intra ocular inflammation which could be due to either an infectious or non-infectious cause. No other disturbances of the iris architecture are apparent.

1. A.

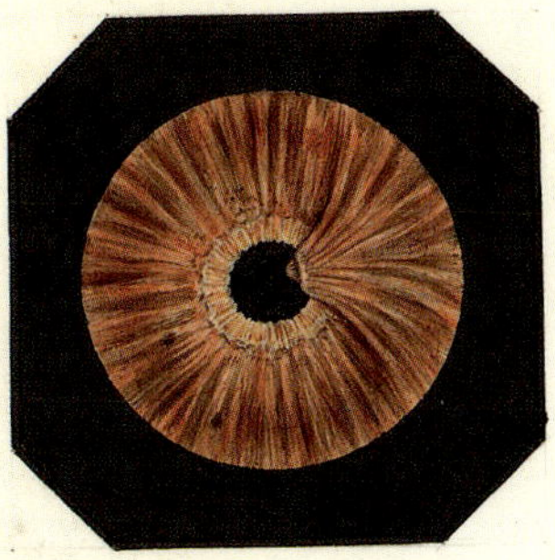

Časanova 3/I 869

Fig. 36
By Dr. Ed. Prochaska 1888

This drawing of a fundus shows several changes. The arterioles are very narrow and there is optic disk whitening. There are large and smaller exudates, with some of the lesions being large drusen. In addition, the retinal pigment epithelium appears to be disturbed. This would appear to be an old central retinal vein occlusion in probably an hypertensive individual. The large exudates would be the residual of such a problem. Alternatively this could be a case of retinitis pigmentosa with large drusen in the posterior pole of the ocular fundus.

Dr. Nussenblatt contributed to this book in his personal capacity. The views expressed are his own and do not necessarily represent the views of the National Institutes of Health or the United States Government.

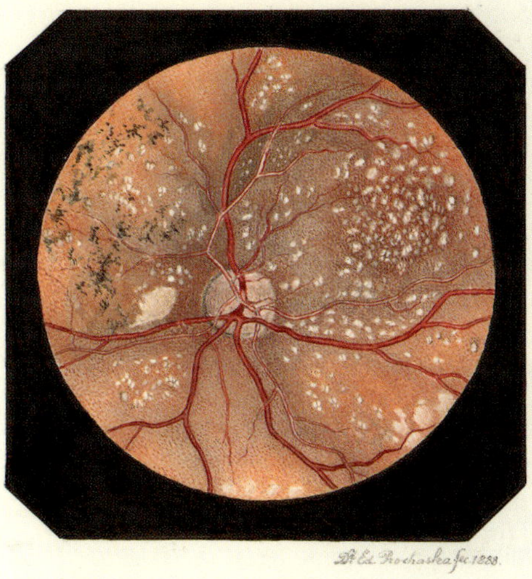
Dr. Ed. Prochaska fec 1883.

Fig. 38
By Dr. Carl Heitzmann 1864

The artist shows an inflamed right eye of a male (?) adult with a large, minimally pigmented mass in the lower temporal fornix reaching up to the 9 o'clock meridian and covering part of the temporal lower quadrant of the cornea also. This might be an inflamed epibulbar dermoid, or possibly a minimally pigmented lesion of conjunctival origin, e.g., a malignant melanoma.

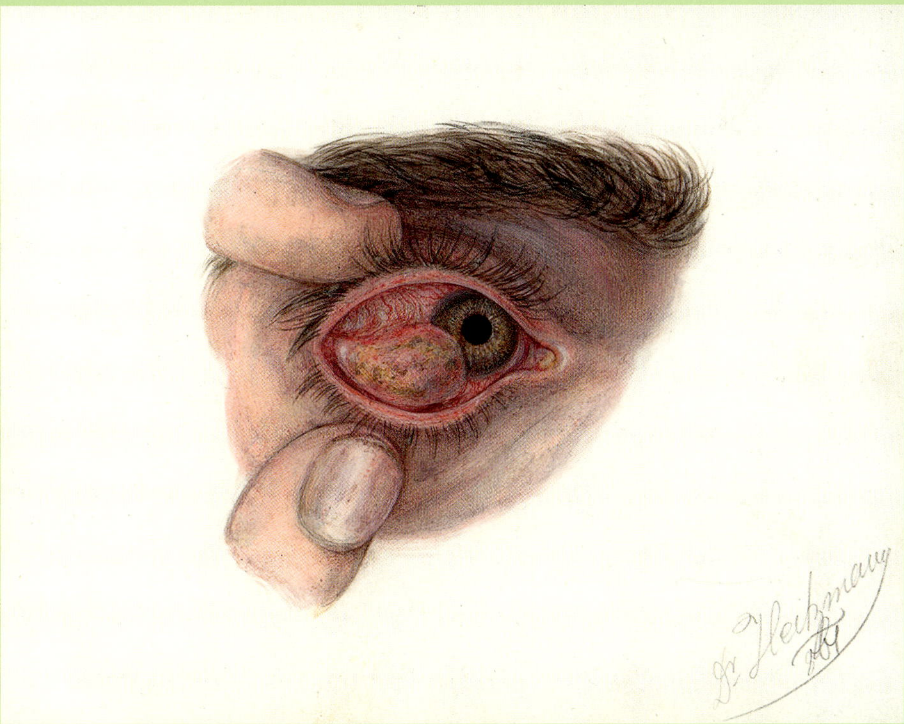

Fig. 39
By Carl Heitzmann 1861

The same artist who painted picture Fig. 38 depicts the right eye of an old male (?) patient with nasal and temporal pinguecula, a prominent gerontoxon and a clear case of cortical and nuclear cataract.

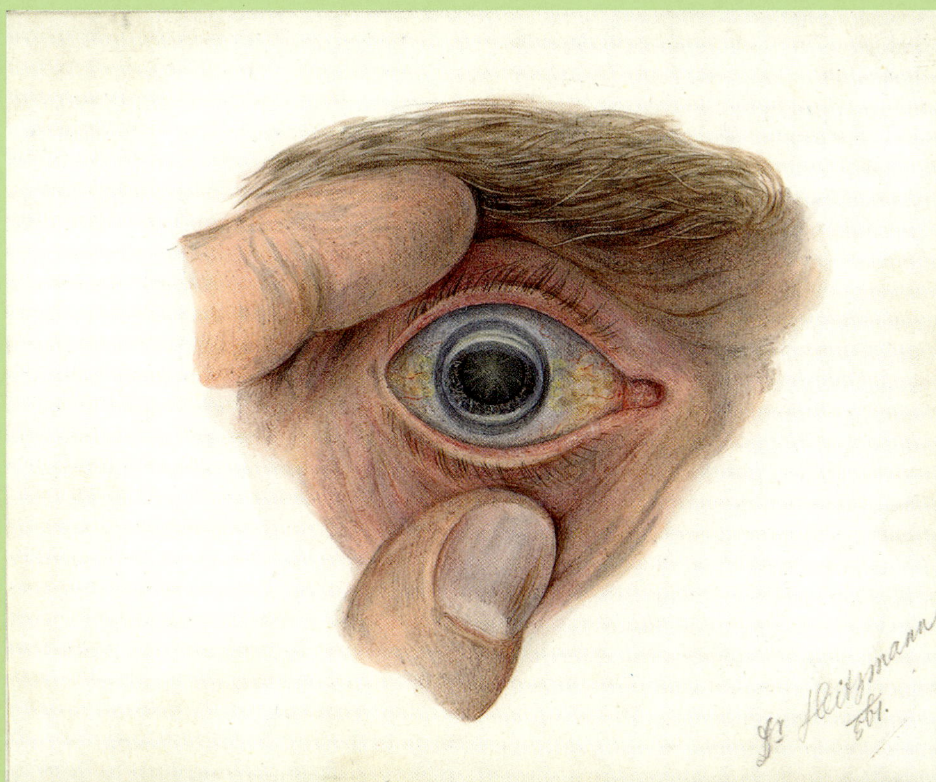

Figs. 40, 41 (Duplicate of Fig. 40)
This is marked as depicting the eyes of a 26 year old farmer's lady with bilateral coloboma of the iris. The other parts of the anterior segments appear to be normal. As these congenital iris colobomata are not located in the usual direction (nasaly inferior) this might also be a case of Rieger's anomaly.

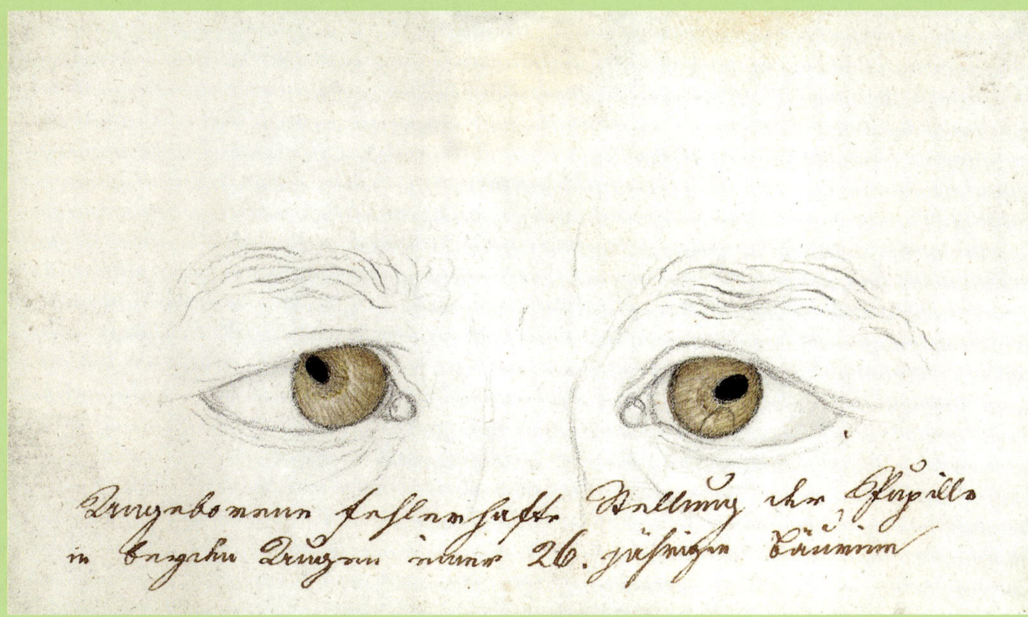

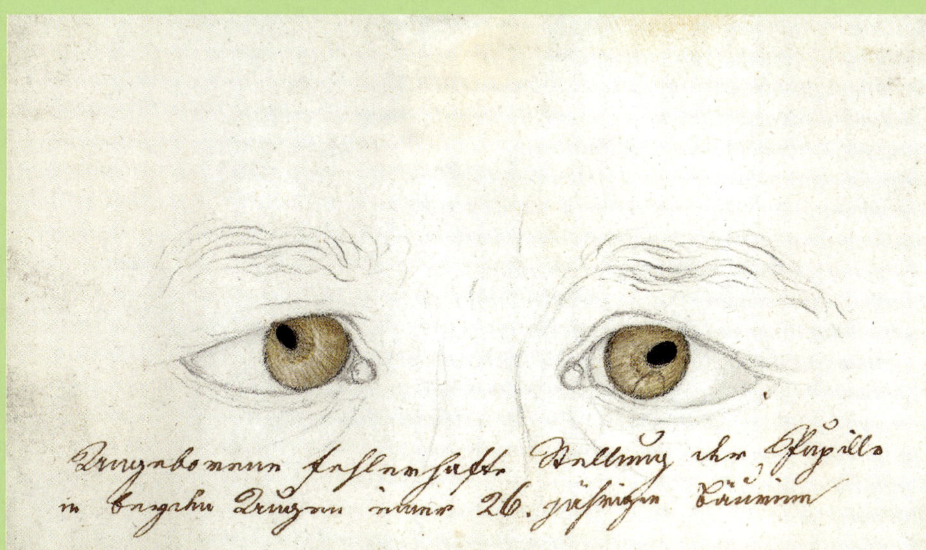

Fig. 42
By Dr. Carl Heitzmann 1867 (Duplicate of Fig. 34)

This patient demonstrates a broad anterior symblepharon from the inner surface of the upper eye lid towards the centre of the cornea where a large nodular mass engulfs most of the surface. It leaves about 2/3 of the limbal area apparently unaffected, although the conjunctiva is definitely shown to be inflamed. The lid margins are inflamed but seem to have a normal structure. This is a rare condition, most probably of limbal origin (tumor-like growth towards the centre ?), but a trauma or an inflammatory cause cannot definitely be ruled out.

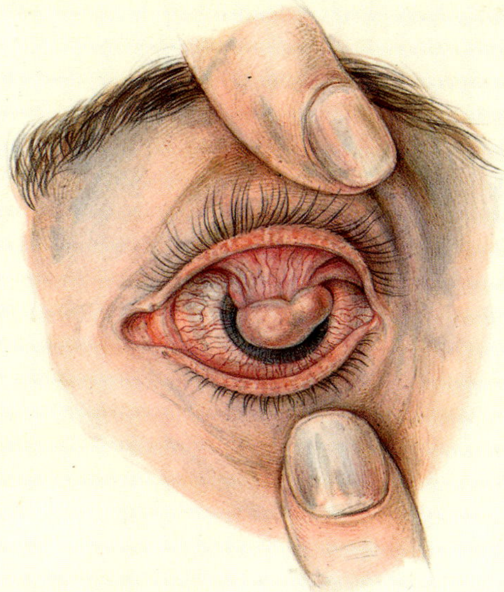

Grimm Julia 8t. Nov. 867.

Fig. 43
By Dr. Georg Joseph Beer 1814/1815

The caption of this painting gives the correct diagnosis: an anterior subcapsular cataract (in this case bilateral and partial) that is associated with atopic dermatitis (post Keratonixydem orta?). The shape of the anterior opacification of the lens is interesting, with both eyes having more dense material apparently on the left hand side and the pupil being widely dilated. At first glance one could assume that a slit-lamp beam had illuminated both lenses from the right, which clearly cannot be the case, as it was painted in 1814/1815.

Cataracta capsularis anterior partialis, post Keratonixydem orta.

Ad No $\frac{175}{2.}$ anno $\frac{1814}{1815}$.

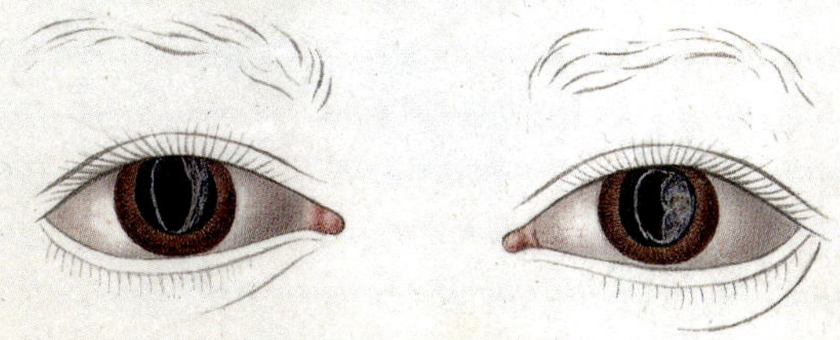

Prof. Beer ad n. p.

Fig. 45
This painting shows a bland left eye with a clear, unaffected cornea and a fleshy mass in the nasal lower quadrant of the anterior chamber. It covers about half of the small pupil and seems to rest on a shallow (3 mm) hyphaema, probably arising from the vascularized tumor. It is slightly pigmented so that the possibility of a ciliary body or iris malignant melanoma comes to mind.

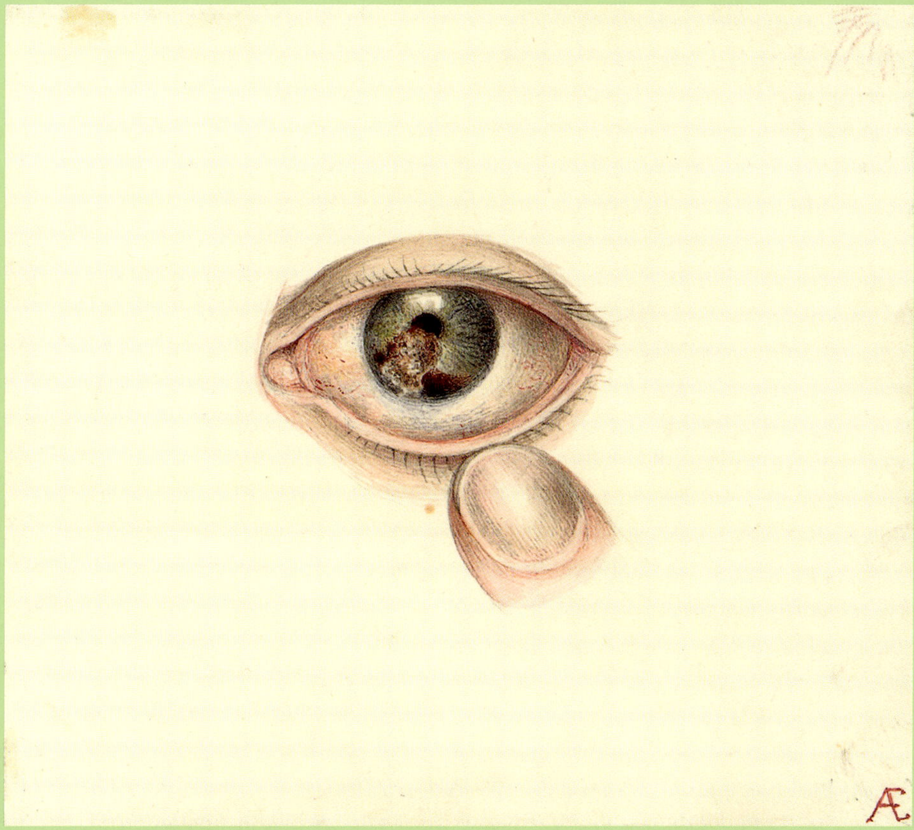
Æ

Fig. 46
By Dr. Georg Joseph Beer

This drawing in profile of the right eye, forehead and nose of a – probably young – man demonstrates a nodular tumor that mildly enlarges the palpebral fissure. It completely covers the cornea, but leaves some aspects of the temporal sclera free. The origin may either be the lid or the conjunctiva/orbit and a diagnosis of a haemangioma can tentatively be made.

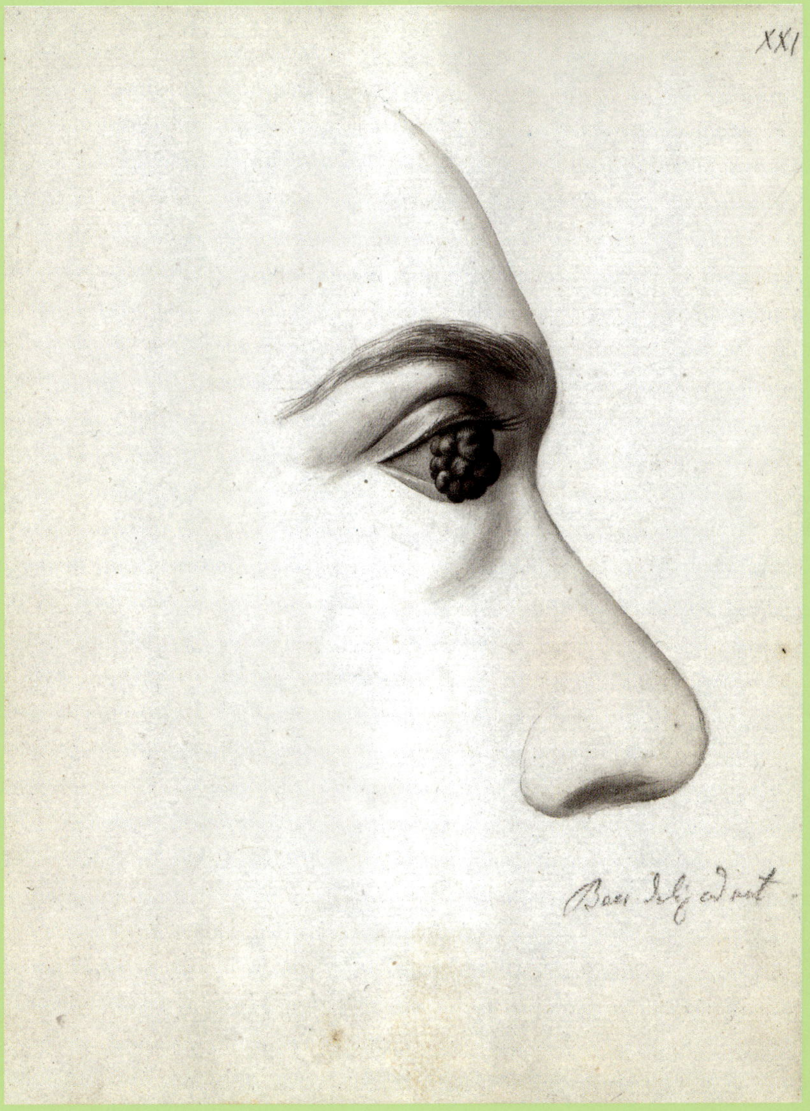
XXI

Fig. 47
By Jos. Zehner 1831/1832

This pencil drawing - or possibly engraving - shows the upper part of a human skull from the left side (with the cranium missing, possibly to study the intracranial extension) with an osseous tumour that fills a large portion of the left orbit. It seems to originate from the roof of the orbit, appears behind the zygomatic bone in the temporal fossa and covers the superior orbital fissure and all but the lower part of the inferior orbital fissure. This could represent an osteoma originating from the frontal or ethmoid sinus with the specimen being prepared by maceration.

This picture corresponds to Fig. 23 by the same artist, described by Robert Nussenblatt, depicting the open skull from above.

VI a)

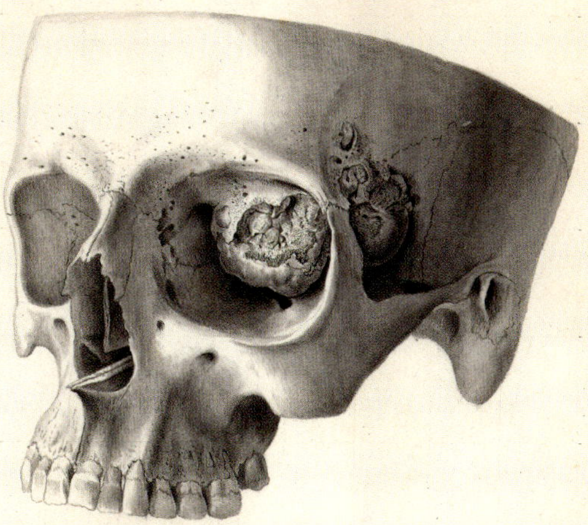

Exostosis orbita
Protocollirt im Schuljahr 1831/32 No 23.

No 23.

Jos. Zehner.

Fig. 48
By Dr. Ed. Prochaska 1888

These early fundus paintings show an atrophic optic nerve head following an (arterial) perivasculitis with narrowing and apparently complete occlusion of the major branches of the central retinal artery of a right eye with possibly few drusen or hard exsudates in the macular area (left picture).

The right picture shows a left fundus with a large tortuous venous vessel in the lower temporal quadrant, possibly following an old branch retinal vein occlusion.

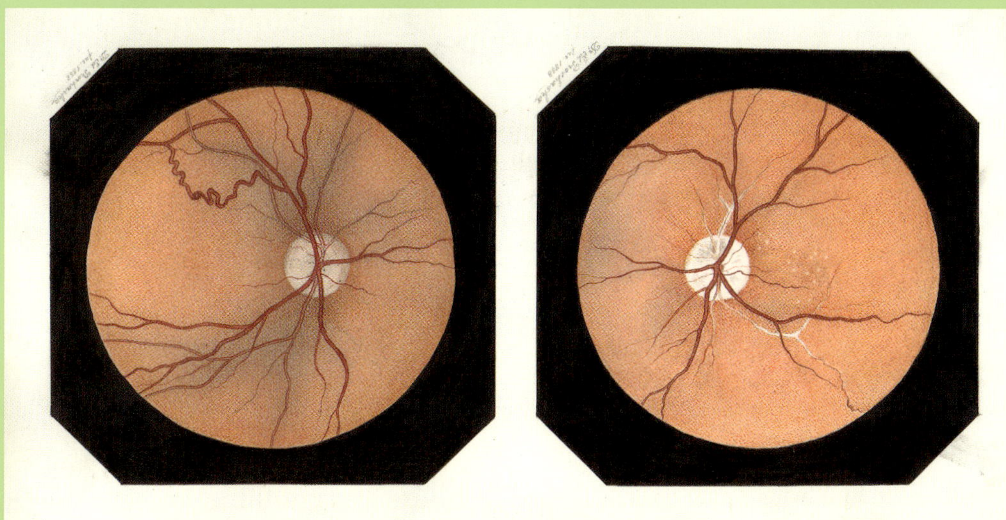

Fig. 49
By Dr. von Celińsky, Warsaw 1833

This intriguing painting shows a patient with unilateral (?), probably conjunctival, multiple reddish nodules mostly in the temporal and superior half (reaching into the medial portion) of the mildly inflamed conjunctiva bulbi. It is unclear whether the blueish hue of the sclera shown is artistic liberty or has any clinical background. The half of the cornea and iris that are depicted appear normal, with probably no inflammation of the anterior segment present. These nodules are not really typical for those observed in sarcoidosis or vernal conjunctivitis, but the red lid margin might point into the later direction if the artist tried to show an everted upper eye lid.

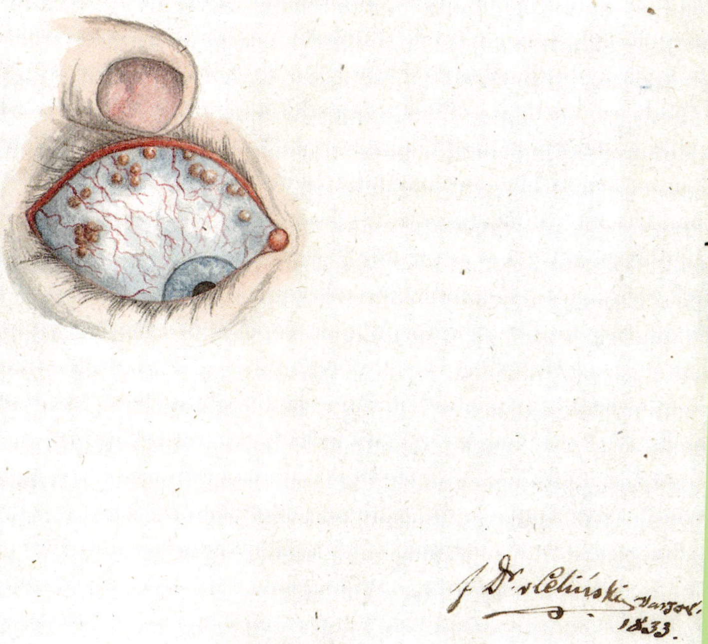
f. Dr. v. Celinski
1833.

Fig. 51

By Dr. Henricus Adelmann, Wirseburg 1843

This is probably a younger patient (possibly in the teens). From the shape of the supercil-iae and the upper lids (mild epicanthus ?) we can suspect that this is a case of Down's syndrome (trisomy 21) and that the upper lid of the left eye is lifted by the examiner to demonstrate the changes of the cornea in an otherwise uninflamed eye. There is no scarring of the cornea shown, but the shape of the red reflex depicted points to a well-developed keratoconus, a corneal condition that is known to be quite frequently associated with this syndrome.

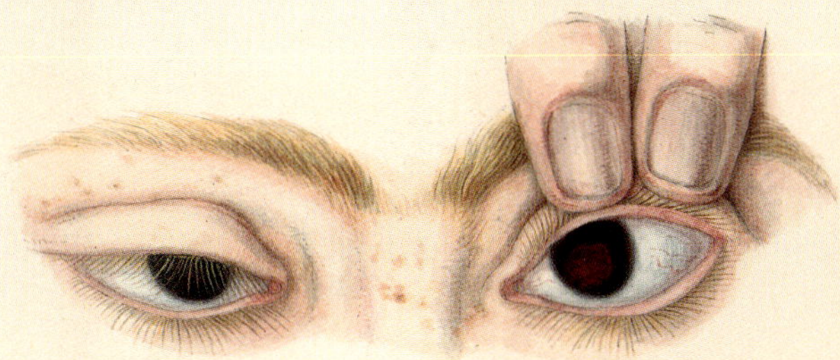

Dr Henricus Adelmann ad naturam pinxit Wirceburgi 1834.

Fig.52
By Dr. Schlossarek 1847

This younger girl (probably in the early to mid-teens) looks complacent, if not really happy to the right side of the observer/painter, probably with only mild pain from the inflamed and enlarged right eye that most certainly has lost sight completely (the left eye shows no signs of anterior segment pathology). This is a long-standing condition, as not only the orbit seems to be enlarged, but also the lids are shown elongated and the palpebral fissure is also significantly greater than on the other side. This points to a quite early onset of the unilateral disease in the first years of life, probably congenital or very early onset glaucoma with secondary inflammation (as shown by a single posterior synechia at the 8:30 position). Amazingly the cornea seems to be clear and regular, although enlarged as in glaucoma, the pupil is widely dilated, the lens seems to be opaque and possibly intumescent.

Fungus medull. oc. d. incipiens. XIV. a.

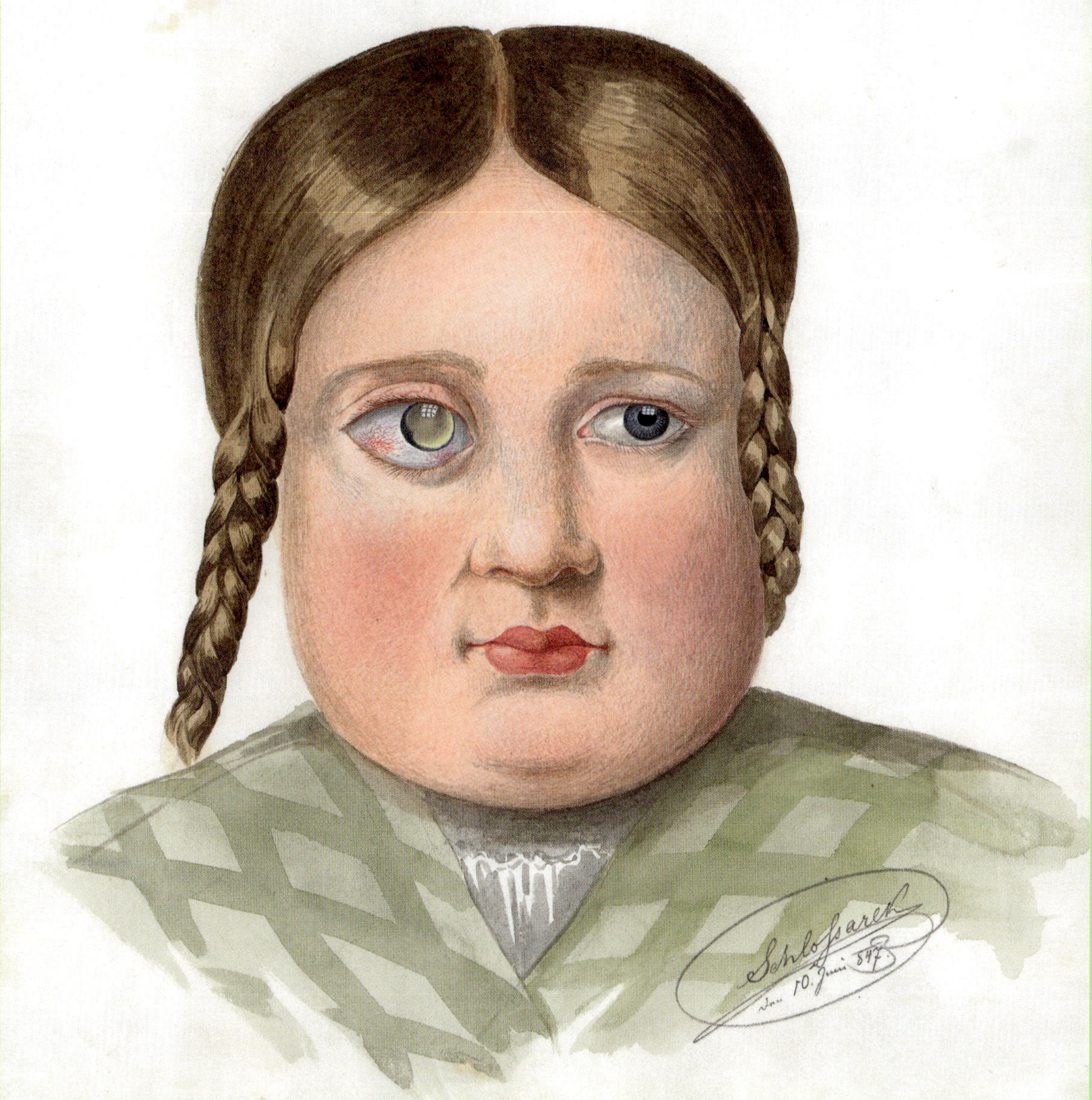

Description by Hans Slezak, ophthalmologist

Fig. 53
By Dr. Máday

The picture shows the head of a man in his fifties. A globular, rather well demarcated tumour protrudes from the upper part of the right orbita, displacing the eye bulb in the lower right direction. The clinical suggestion points to a benign mixed tumour of the lachrymal gland. The displacement of the eye without major involvement of the morphology of the eye lids constitutes a characteristic symptom of this neoplasm.

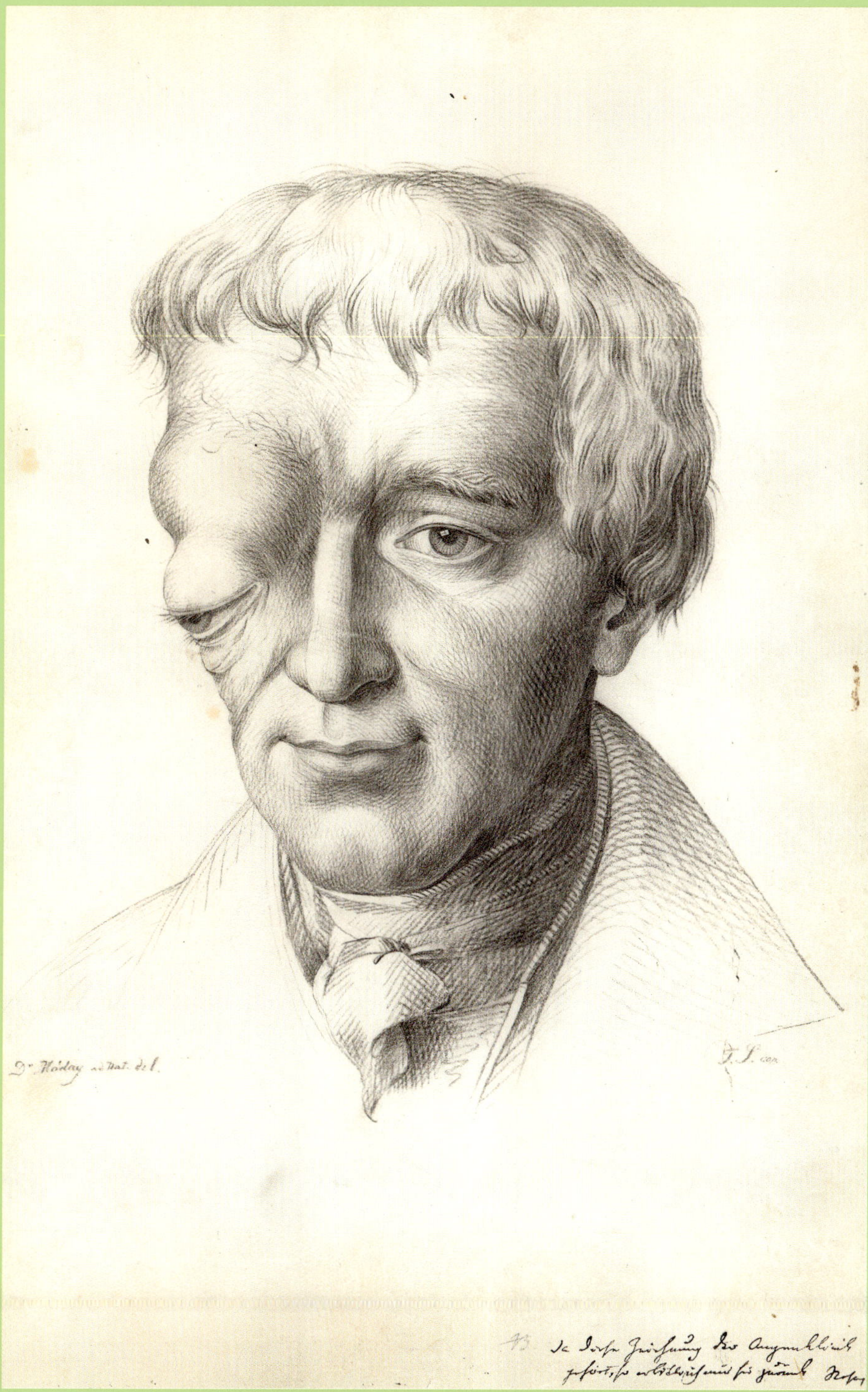

Fig. 54
By Dr. Máday

Same patient, obviously after successful enucleation of the tumour by transpalpebral orbitotomia.

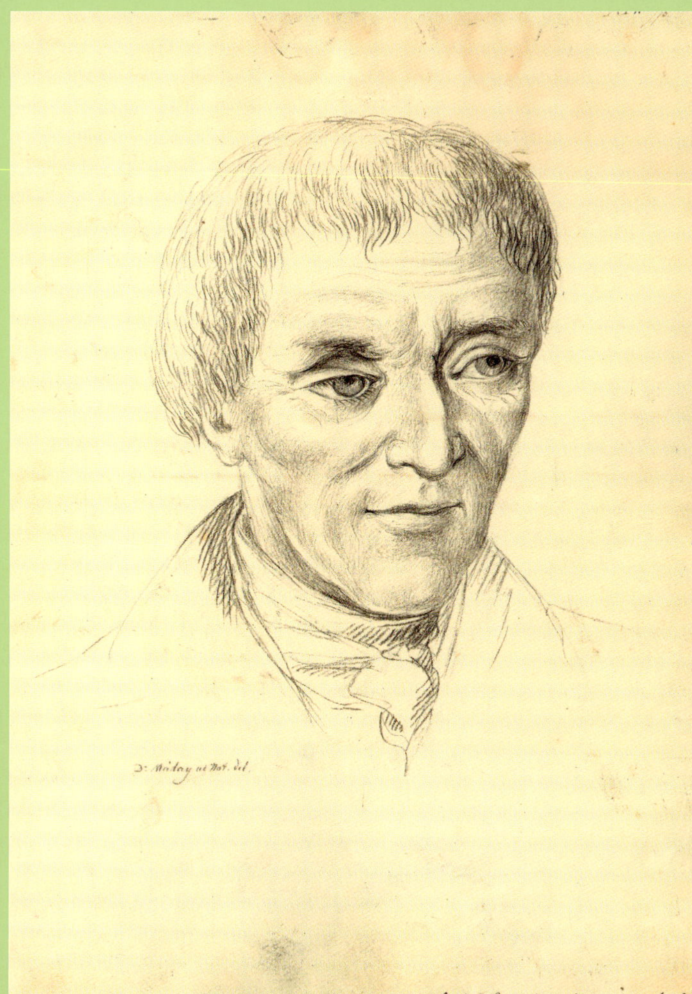

Description by Anselm Kampik ophthalmologist and ophthalmo-pathologist

Fig. 55 a–c
By Dr. Otto Pecker and Dr. Carl Heitzmann

A treatise in Medizinische Jahrbücher volume XIII, 1867, by Otto Becker and Vinzenz Czerny, deals with eye diseases treated at the University of Vienna during the years 1863–1865, of which we have the original histopathology pictures some of which were published in the above article. Here a modern commentary is presented.

Then as much as today, the adenoid of the lachrymal gland is a rare disease. Relation to the report by Rothmund jr. is made, who founded the present-day department of ophthalmology at Mathilden-Strasse in Munich.

The pictures of Fig. 55 a–f demonstrate with exemplary precision the classical characteristics of this adenoid of the lachrymal gland. Modern histopathology reports cannot match the pictures of yesteryear and photography of today could not do better. Sketchy presentation of the salient features is a hallmark of the images.

Fig. 55 a demonstrates the separation of normal glandular tissue from the adenoid by layers of connective tissue whereas Fig. 55 c illustrates the infiltrative growth of the tumour into formations of normal glandular tissue.

Colloid material and alveolar-like structures are depicted in Figs. 55 b and, magnified, in Figs. 55 d, e, f.

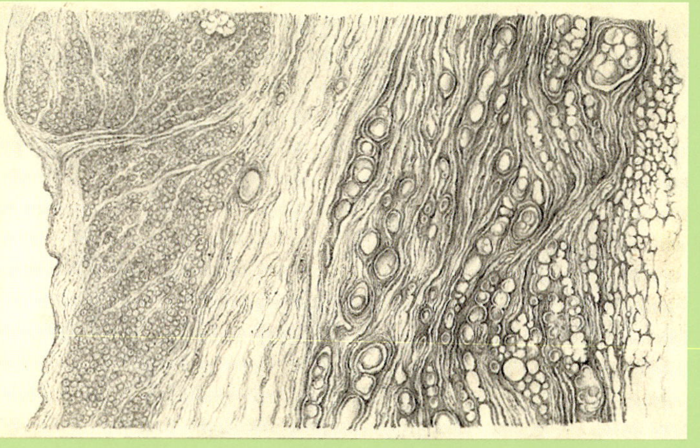

a

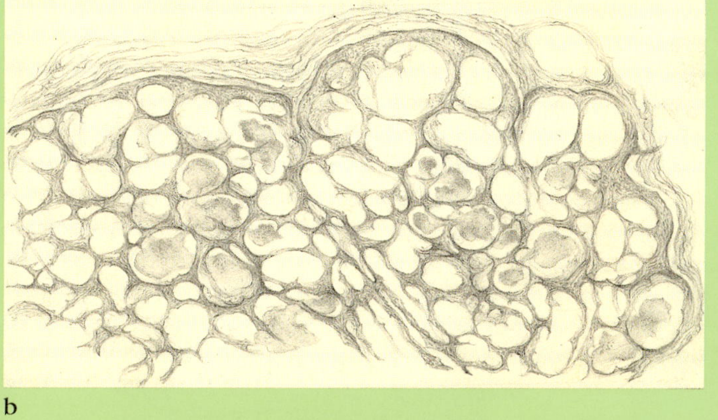

b

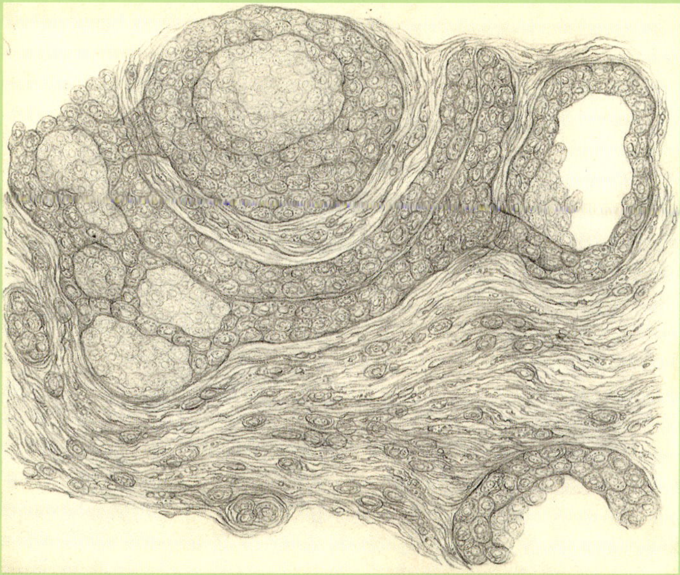

c

Figs. 56
Figs. 57
Figs. 58
all by Dr. Vinzenz Czerny and Dr. Carl Heitzmann

Sympathic ophthalmia

Czerny stated in the above article: "Still we are at the beginning of all considerations of how the lesion of one eye, sadly, results in a concomitant (sympathetic) involvement of the other eye."

Even the most detailed histopathologic investigations did not lead anywhere. The drawings depict granulomatous inflammation and its consequences, the involvement of ciliary nerves and the formation of tumour like proliferations with multinucleated cells.

Even on the basis of exact observations no explanation could be deduced then, of the aetiology of sympathic ophthalmia. More than a century passed before immunology lead the way to the discovery of its mechanisms targeting retinal tissue.

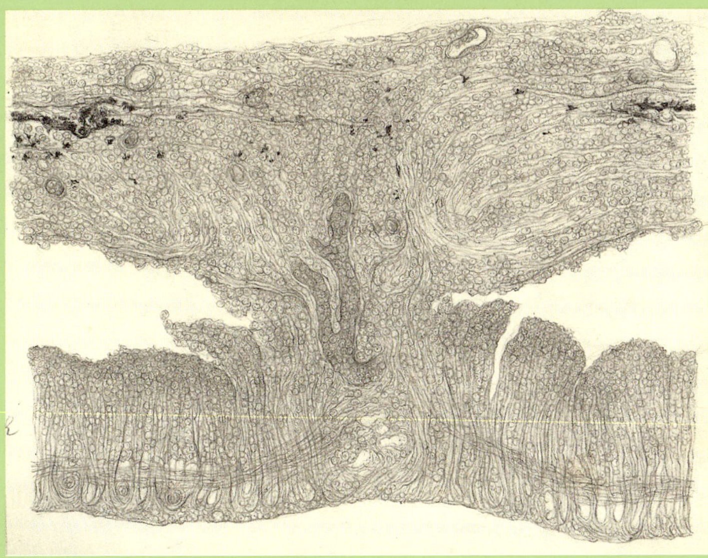
56

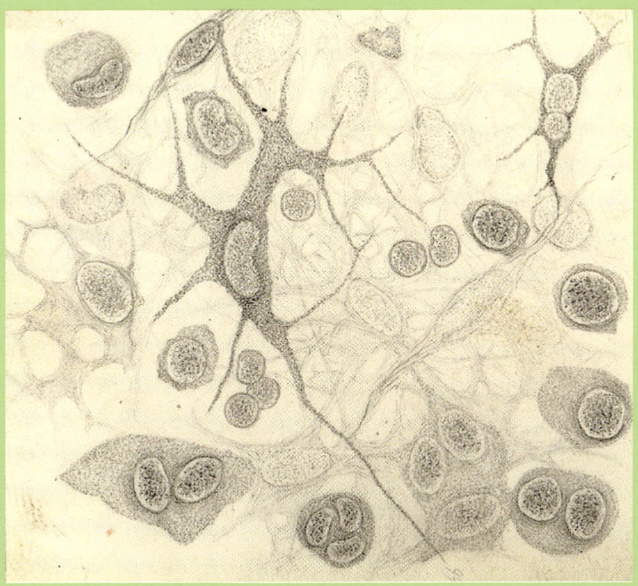
57

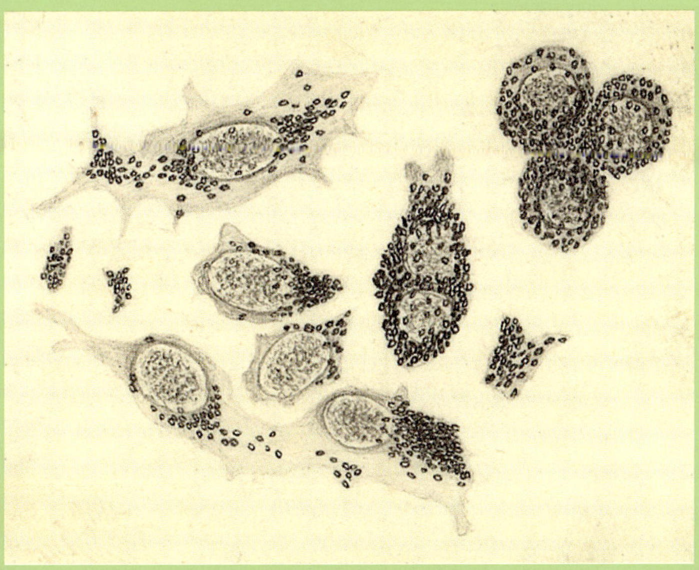
58

Figs. 59 a–c
Staphyloma corneae

Function of the cornea as main lens of the eye is guaranteed only by continuous maturation and regeneration of its epithelium, which thereby, remains an important field of study. Understandably, this lead to speculations as to its derivation. Today the discovery and knowledge of the nature of stem cells has clarified much. 130-odd years ago this was unknown and the theory of a derivation of epithelial from connective tissue cells was rampant.

How relative are discussions, how much do they depend on theories of the time!

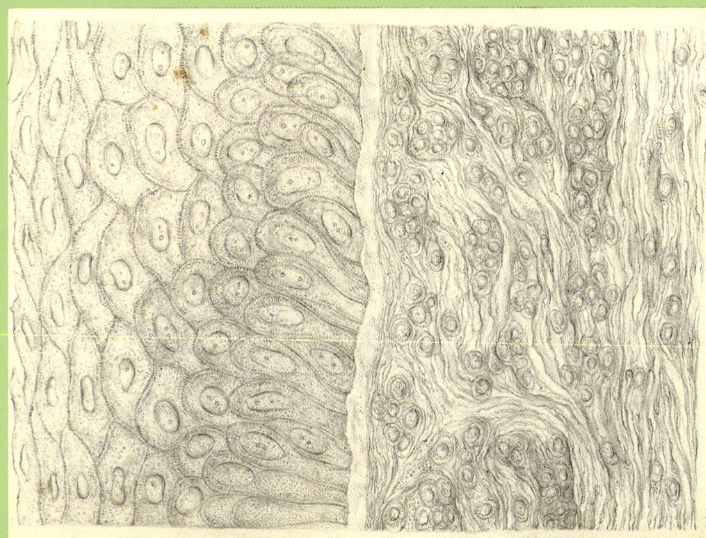

a

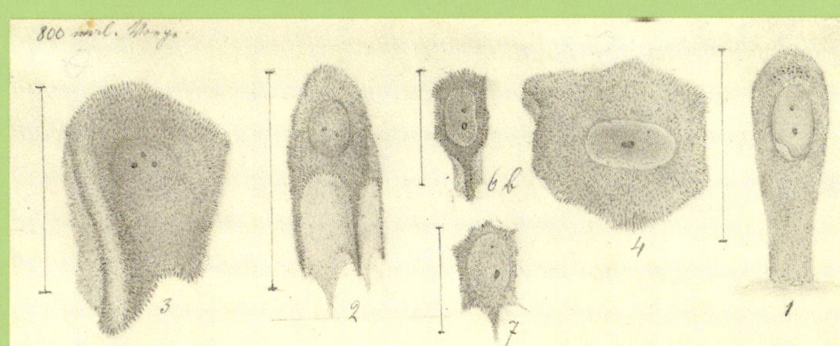

b

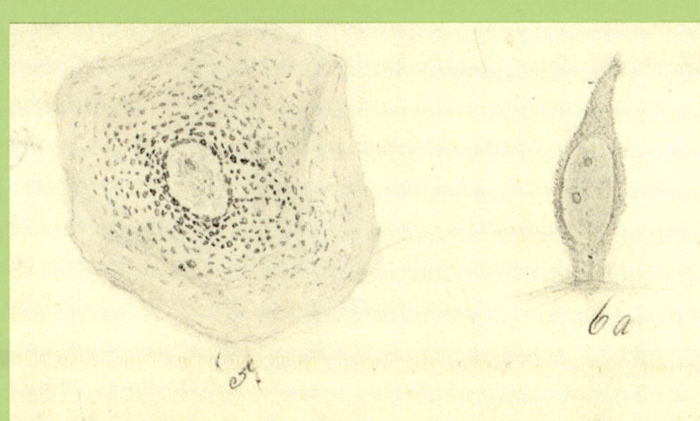

c

Description by Peter Propping, geneticist

Fig. 60
By Parlianz 1887

Girl with Neuroma multiforme
The drawing shows a poor girl of perhaps five years with a monstrous mass of the upper left eyelid. The whole eyelid consists of a tumour that draws the eyebrow downward and covers the eye completely as well as major parts of the cheek. Only some eyelashes at the medial side remind the viewer that the massive tumour is what used to be an upper lid. The situation is even more grotesque because the tumour like a parasite dominates not only an otherwise lovely face of a suffering girl but is also a threat to her young life.

The term neuroma, i. e., a schwannoma is sometimes falsely used for a neurofibroma. It is likely that the depicted tumour is a neurofibroma plexiforme that may occur in the context of the autosomal dominant neurofibromatosis 1 (NF1) von Recklinghausen. Since the face of the girl does not present additional signs of a neurofibromatosis, the tumour may also be sporadic. In any case it developed from a cell clone in which the two copies of the tumour suppressor gene NF1 are mutated. The innocent girl who hardly knows her future reminds us of the vulnerability of our genes and the devastating consequences of mutations.

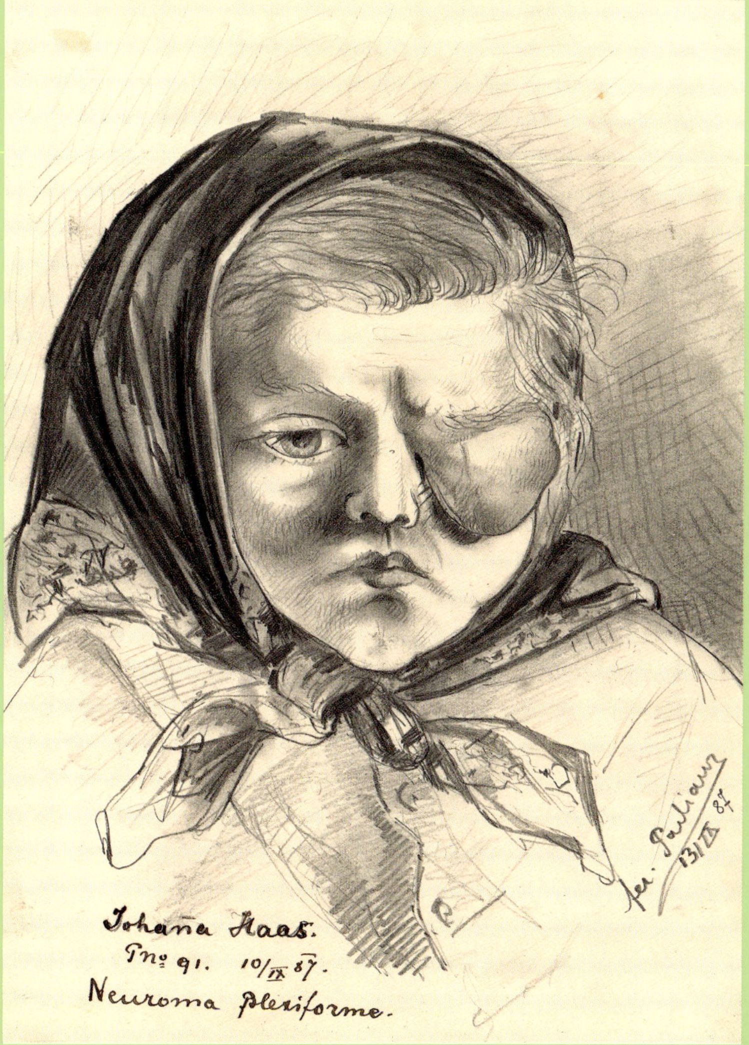
Johaña Haas.
Pno 91. 10/IX 87.
Neuroma plexiforme.
fec. Galiauz
13/IX 87

Jörg-Christian Tonn, neurosurgeon

Fig. 62
By Gartner 1845

The person on the drawing shows an exophthalmus on the right side with visible signs of compression. The eyeball is not only markedly protruding, there is also an extensive edema of the upper and lower eyelid. Despite the considerable swelling of the lids, which normally would lead to complete closure of the eye, the exophthalmus is so monstrous that the eyeball is pushing the lids open. Well recognizable is a swelling in the area of the conjunctiva. The pupil, as compared to the healthy left side, is of the same width, the eye due to the malposition seems to be gazing.

Differential diagnoses of the disease as shown in the figure range from arteriovenous fistula of the cavernous sinus and thrombosis of the cavernous sinus to intraconal retroorbital tumour. A pulsating whirring when palpating the bulging eyeball or auscultation with the stethoscope (with a pulse synchronous, machine like noise) would lead almost with certainty to the diagnosis of cavernous sinus fistula without further measures. Today magnetic resonance techniques and CT scans enable the physician to come to a rapid diagnosis. The AV fistula in the cavernous sinus, the (painful) thrombosis of the cavernous sinus or any compression due to retroorbital infection or retroorbital tumour – they all can be depicted rapidly and reliably with the use of the additional imaging techniques. Appropriate therapy could be administered without delay. The protrusion as shown on the drawing with the extensive venous compression does not only represent a cosmetic problem, it also bears a functional danger for the visual acuity of the right eye since visual loss is threatening rapidly. In case of carotid cavernous sinus fistula, today special catheter systems can elegantly be advanced endovascularly to the fistula via puncture of the inguinal artery. With the use of appropriate material (balloon systems, platinum wire coils or a combination of both) the fistula can be closed selectively. In case of tumour growth microsurgical operations or targeted stereotactic single session radiation (radiosurgical therapy) as well as a combination of the latter two are remedial measures. The way from at-a-glance-diagnosis of this impressive lesion to its specific treatment today can be very short.

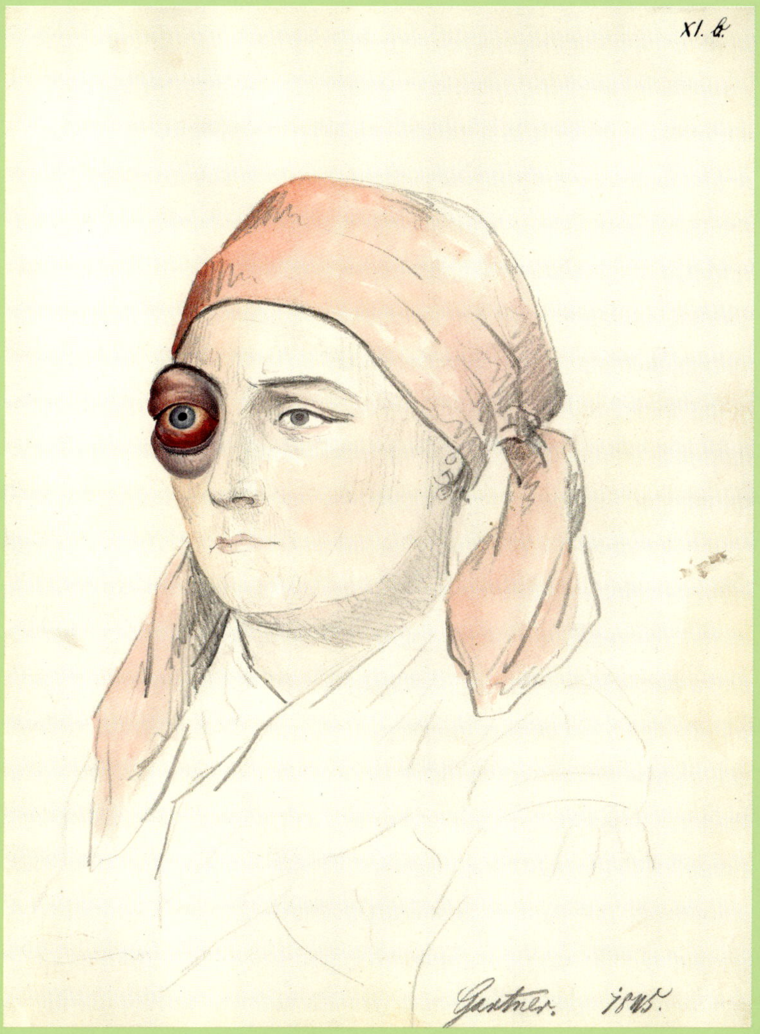
XI. 6.
Gastner. 1845.

Fig. 63, by an unknown painter
1832/1833

The person shown on the drawing is suffering from ptosis, i.e., sagging of the upper eyelid on the right side. Furthermore there is obviously a slight protrusion of the eye which appears to be directed outside/down. Furthermore the pupil, just to be seen at the border, is distinctly enlarged as compared with the healthy left side. On the drawing the diagnosis Exophthalmus a tumore cystico orbitae has been written down. First of all the drawing impresses by both an inner (concerning the pupil) and outer (affecting the position of bulbus and eyelid opening) oculomotor paresis. Causes of such symptoms may be multiple. Most frequent are intra- or retroorbital tumours, not seldom also sphenoid-ridge meningiomas with participation of the cavernous sinus or solely meningiomas in the cavernous sinus. Also it could be a paralytic aneurysma of the carotid artery which, especially in the region of the posterior communicating artery, would damage the oculomotor nerve through direct compression. For an aneurysmatic genesis an exophthalmus would be non-typic, however, on the drawing the exophthalmus does not seem to be in the foreground. These two most frequent differential diagnoses can easily be separated by anamnestic data, since disorders of a paralytic aneurysma appear suddenly, in case of tumour, however, insidiously. Certainly also infectious diseases have to be taken into account in a differential diagnosis. By means of tomographic magnetic imaging (MRI) a number of possibilities could easily be represented or excluded. Since on the present drawing the oculomotor paresis is not yet complete (and prognosis of recovery depends heavily on the duration of the symptoms), implementation of therapeutic measures is urgently required.

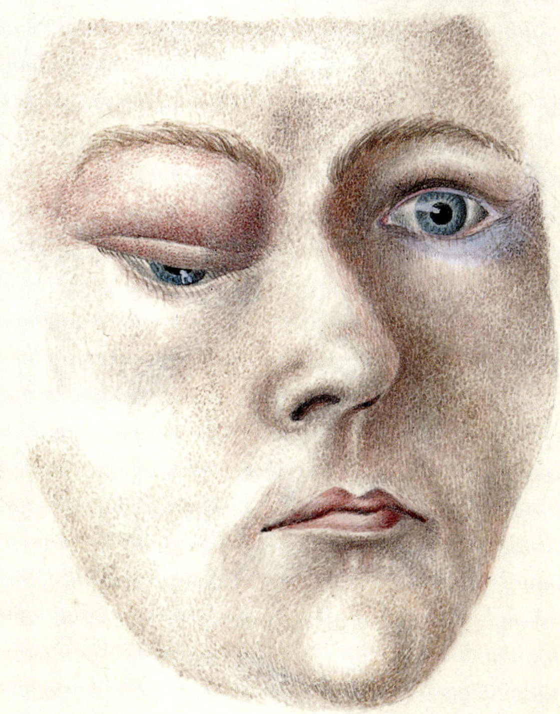

Exophthalmus a tumore cystico orbitæ

Protocoll. 1832/3 N 73.

Description by Wilfred Druml, nephrologist

Fig. 64
By A. Schlossarek 1847

A young lady with a massive swelling of the eye lids. In this age this is most likely due to oedema in the context of a nephrotic syndrome, such as in minimal change nephritis or lupus nephritis (which would explain the red cheeks). Massive lipid accumulation in the eye lids would be another explanation, but this is very unusual at the age of the patient.

Pladaroma palpebrarum. Nro. XVIII.

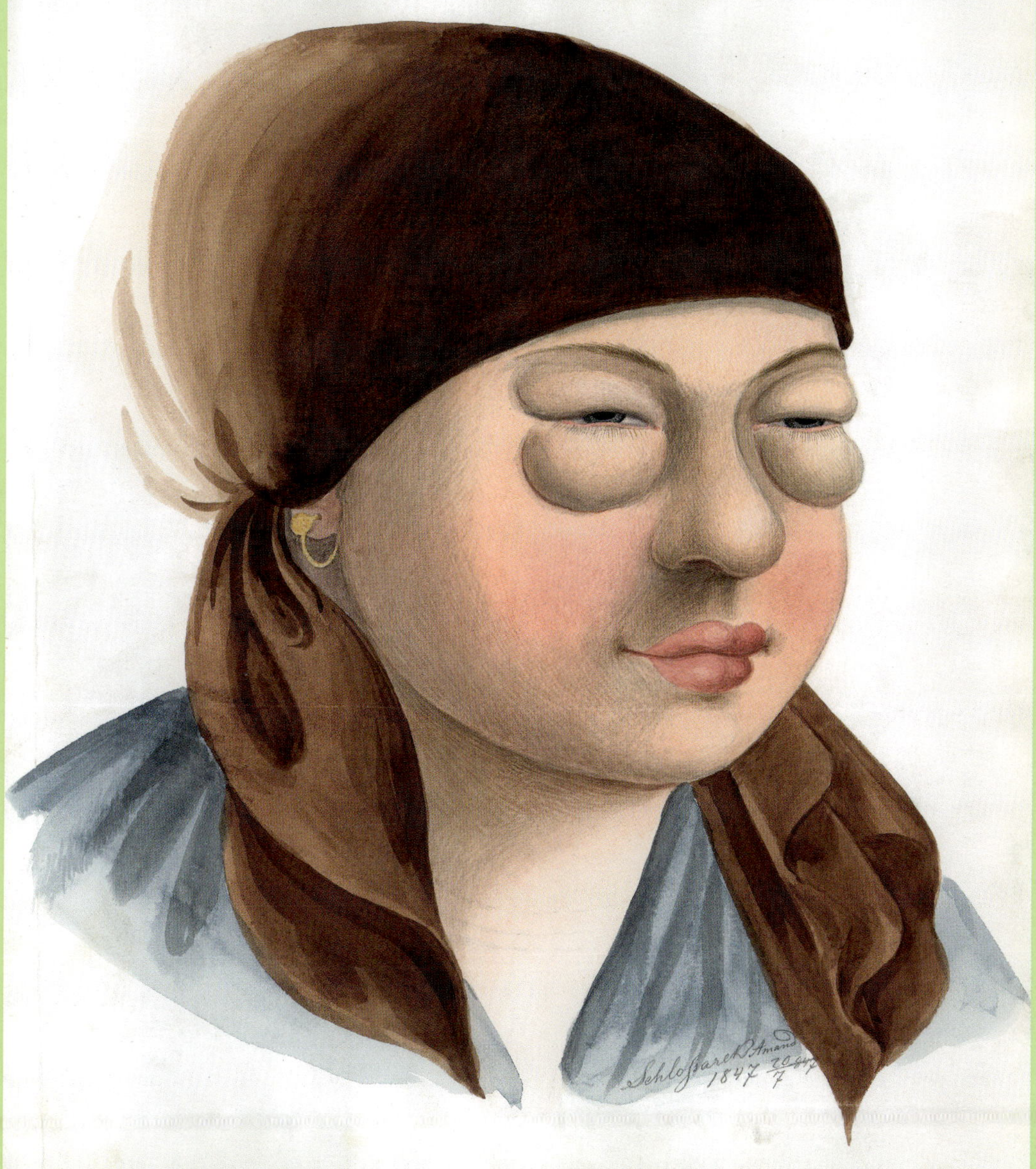

Description by Kurt Jellinger, neuroanatomist

Fig. 65
The following interpretations appear reasonable:

Inscription only partly readable. Picture shows basis of the brain with severely damaged and atrophic right bulb and severe atrophy of the optic tract.
Compare Figs. 23, 47.

TAB.

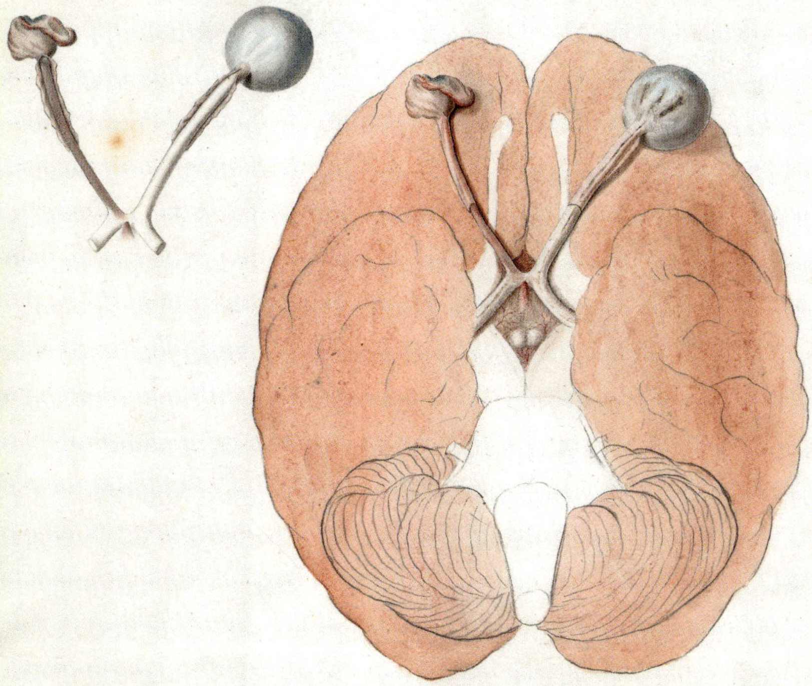

Atrophisches Auge mit seinem atrophischen Sehnerven

Fig. 66
By Dr. Carl von Rzehaczek

Large left frontal tumor (type not classifiable) with invasion of the left orbit and large hemorrhagic and partly necrotic mass in the left orbit.

XIV.

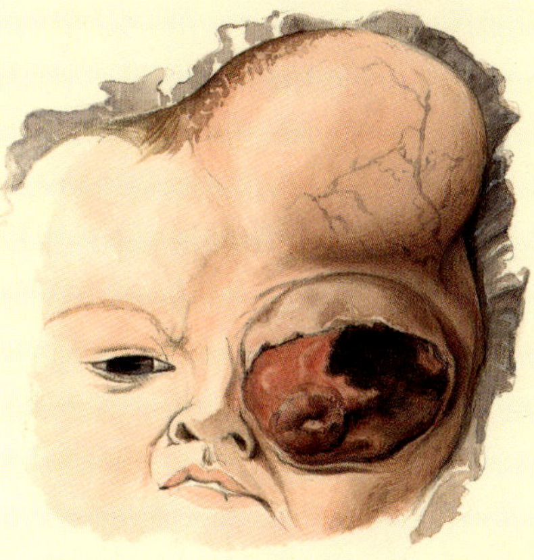

Dr Rzehaczek fecit.

Fig. 68
By Jos. Zehner, 1831/1832

Large fungal mass invading both orbits and anterior fossa as well as anterior parts of the brain.

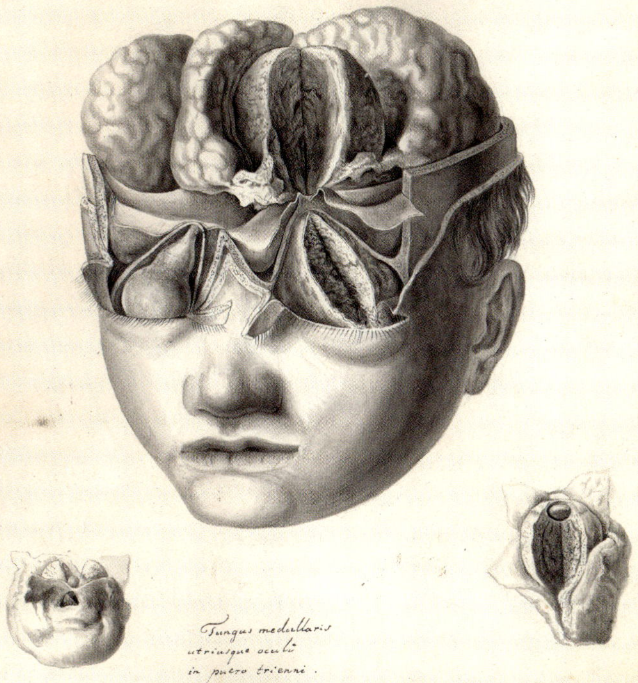

Fungus medullaris
utriusque oculi
in puero trienni.

Protocollirt.
No 41. 18 31/32

Jos. Zehner.
fec. ad nat

Description by Kuniaki Ohara, dermatologist

Fig. 69
By Dr. Anton Elfinger 1862

The geographical scar affects the front and upper eyelid, thus resulting the scar contracture of the eyelid, ectropion. The arborizing or flame-like pattern of a white scar suggests that this patient had suffered from deep dermal or third degree burn in the past. A dotted line illustrates the design of the surgical correction of the contracture by a transposition flap with frontal skin. From the dermatological point of view, it is not advisable to reconstruct the upper eyelid with frontal skin. The thick frontal skin could not substitute the thin, soft and movable eyelid skin. And it is not clearly understood what the crescent line around the lateral side of eyebrow means. The author might intend to replace the damaged eyebrow with lanugos of frontal skin.

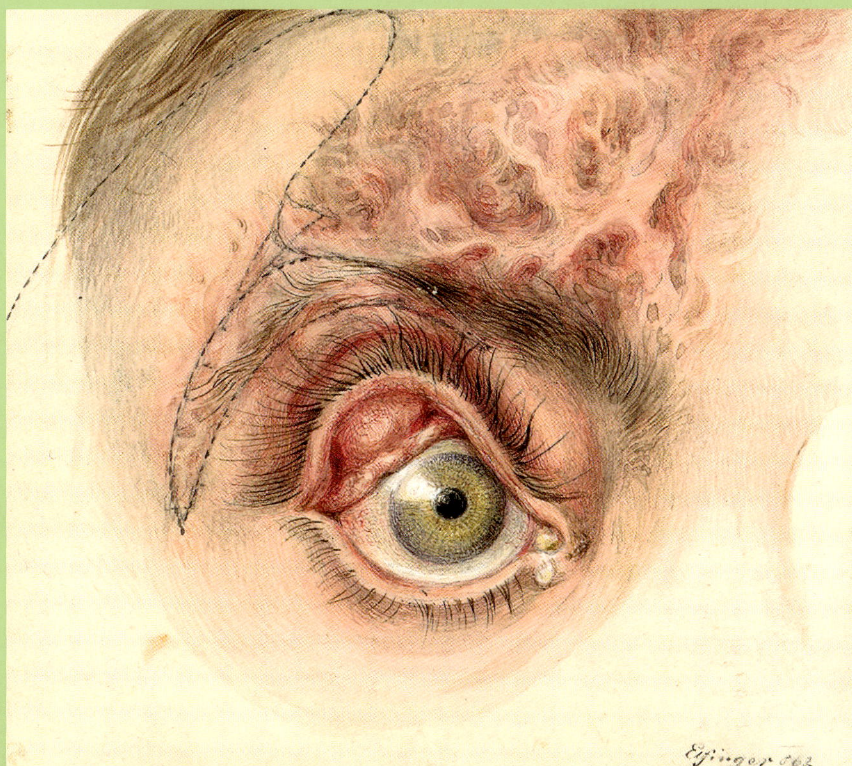

Fig. 70
By Dr. Anton Elfinger 1861

Granulating proliferation is noted on the upper conjunctiva, and the lower eyelid skin is lost in triangular fashion. This skin loss seems to be superficial or partial in thickness, because the lower eyelash is preserved, so the orbicular muscle or tarsal plate is left. Although basal cell carcinoma is the most common skin disease that destroys the lower eyelid, in that situation, full thickness tissue is usually invaded. So the skin loss might be due to dissecting injury or trauma and the change of the upper eyelid might be the result of secondary inflammation. Another possibility is some kind of chronic infection, such as syphilis, tuberculosis or fungus.

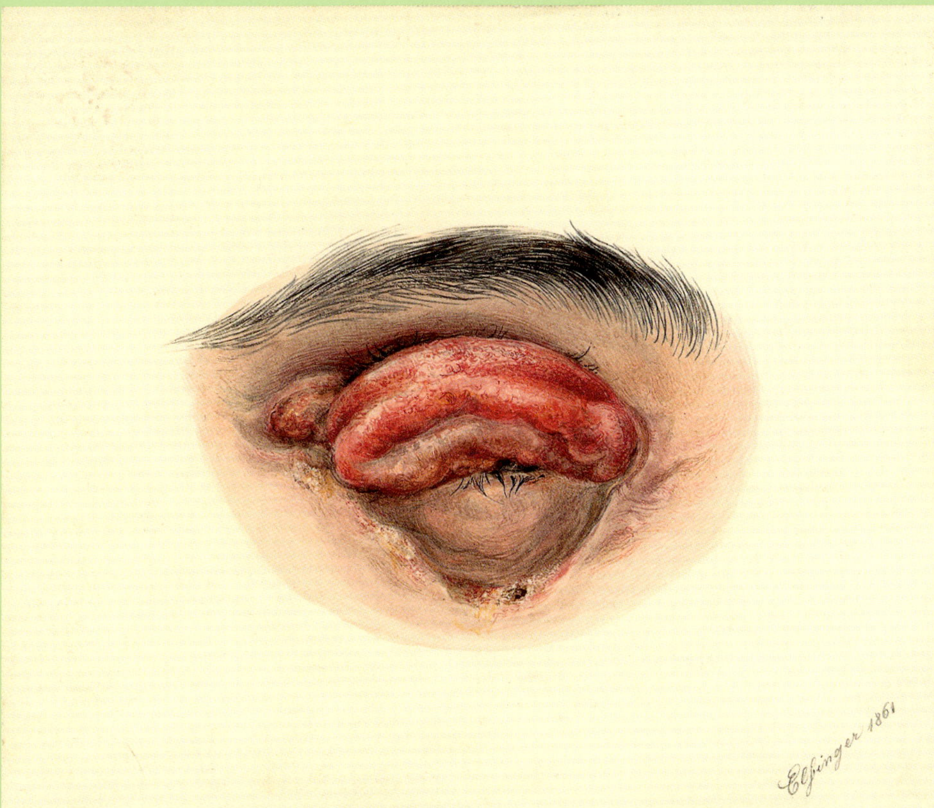
Elfinger 1861

Description by Rudolf Happle, dermatologist

Fig. 71
By Nob(ilis) de Schrötter

The legend reads "The portrait of the travelling white Negro Georg Gamber, whom I presented publicly at the Eye Hospital on 22 January 1813".

The roundel shows an adult man affected with oculo-cutaneous albinism. From the wording "travelling white Negro" we may infer that this man was gaining some money by exposing himself in penny shows at fairs. Needless to say that the term "white Negro" may have attracted public curiosity far more effectively than the sober wording "completely white man" would have done (see also comment on the paintings Figs. 72, 73).

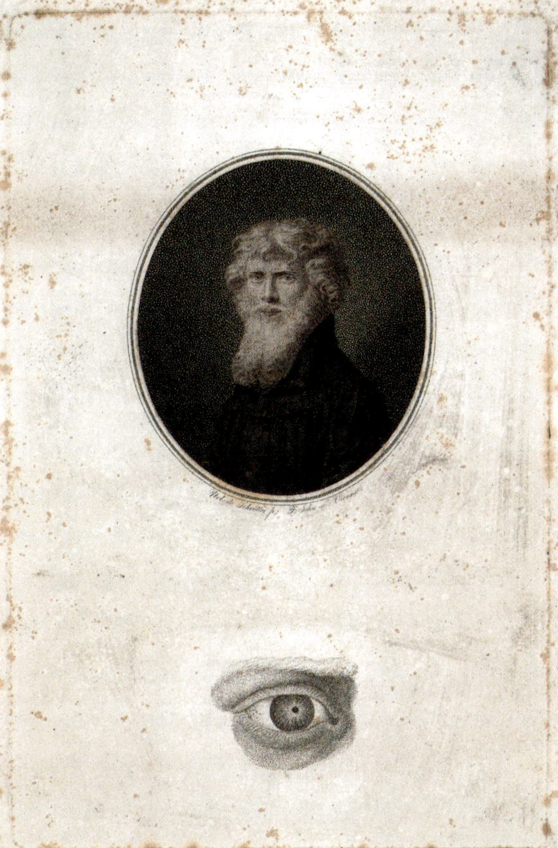

Das Bild des reisenden weißen Mohren Georg Gamber, welchen ich am 12ten Jänner 1810 öffentlich auf der Augenklinik vorzeigte. Beer

Figs. 72, 73
By Dr. Georg Joseph Beer 1814

The legend reads "Iacob Danzinger, a 10-year-old white Negro, born at Her(r)nals near Vienna". Under the roundel picture we read "Prof. Beer p[inxit] 1814".

The two paintings show a boy with oculo-cutaneous albinism. I am inclined to guess that this was a case of tyrosinase positive albinism because the scalp hair, the eyebrows and the lashes seem to contain minimal spots of remaining melanin, which would not be seen in the tyrosinase negative form of oculo-cutaneous albinism.

Nowadays the German expression weisser Mohr (literally: white Moor) is no longer understood. The wording does not mean an albino Negro, nor does it designate an individual of Moorish descent. Rather, this term was used to denote an individual who looked as unusual as a Negro would have looked within the European population of that time, but being completely white instead of black.

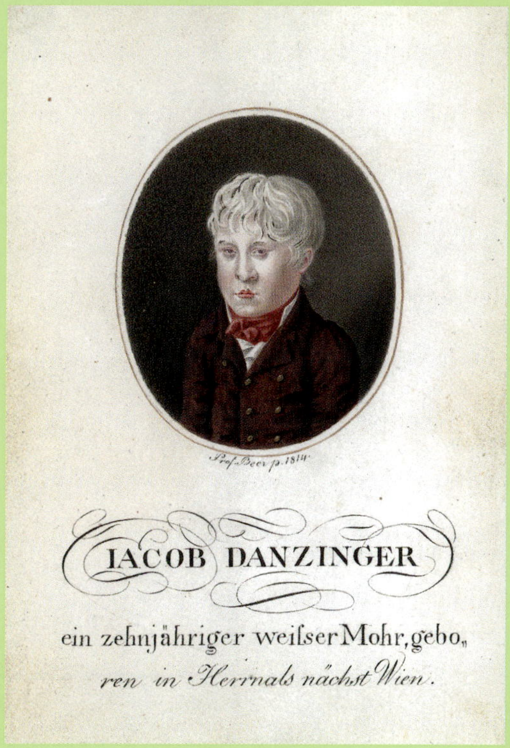
Prof. Beer p. 1814
IACOB DANZINGER
ein zehnjähriger weisser Mohr, gebo„
ren in Herrnals nächst Wien.
72

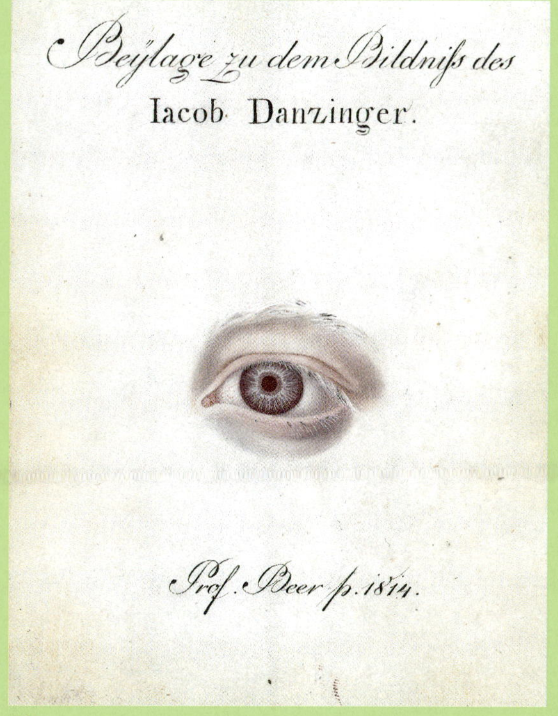
Beylage zu dem Bildniss des
Iacob Danzinger.
Prof. Beer p. 1814.
73

Fig. 74
By Dr. Carl von Rzehaczek 1843

This girl has a large unilateral tumor that has displaced the ipsilateral eye and eyebrow. In 2003 we have argued that this may be a case of plexiform neurofibroma[1]. Today, I should like to add that the sharp perpendicular line of demarcation of the hyperpigmentation as present on the forehead can be taken as an additional argument in favor of this diagnosis.
Hence, this impressive painting most likely shows a tumour reflecting loss of heterozygosity that occurred at an early developmental stage[1]. In other words, this may be an example of a type 2 segmental manifestation of neurofibromatosis 1, documented about 150 years prior to the recognition of this clinico-genetic concept[2].

(1) Happle R, Holubar K: An eye for an eye … (Exodus xxi:23,24). J Invest Dermatol 2003;120:893-894
(2) Happle R: A rule concerning the segmental manifestation of autosomal dominant skin disorders: review of clinical examples providing evidence for dichotomous types of severity. Arch Dermatol 1997;133:1505-1509

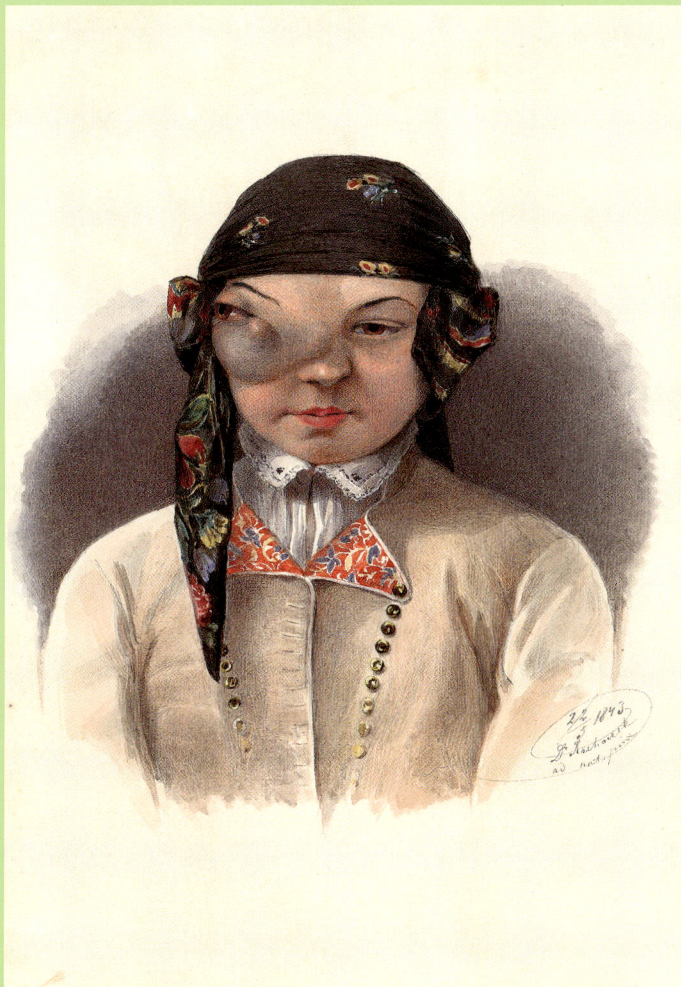

22/5 1843
ad nat. pinx.

Fig. 75
By A. Lindner

At a first glance I had the feeling: Don't make a definite diagnosis in this case! I showed the painting to several colleagues, and some of them described a unilateral atrophy, whereas others saw a unilateral augmentation of tissue. Hence, it is a picture puzzle.

Those seeing an atrophy may think of hemiatrophia faciei progressiva (Romberg syndrome), or of an atypical case of morphea. However, the lateral displacement of the right eye is at variance with these diagnostic possibilities. Those who see a swelling may think of a plexiform neurofibroma. In my view, the best solution is to avoid any specific diagnosis in this case.

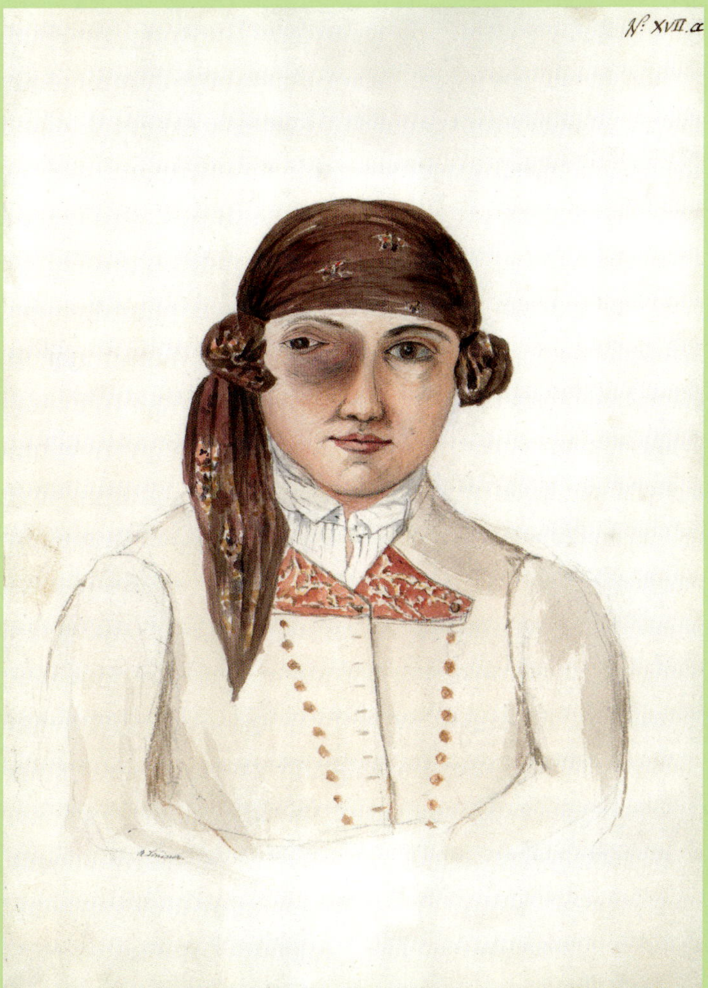
No. XVII.a

Description by Georg Stingl, dermatologist

Fig. 76
By Jos. Zehner 1832/1833

This is obviously the more difficult for a non-ophthalmologist. As opposed to what is written on the original (Caruncula carcinomatodes) I don't believe that this is a malignancy. In view of the obvious mutilations on the nose, I am considering the occurrence of granulomatous processes, syphilitic gumma, granulomas by typical or atypical mycobacteria etc.

A IX:

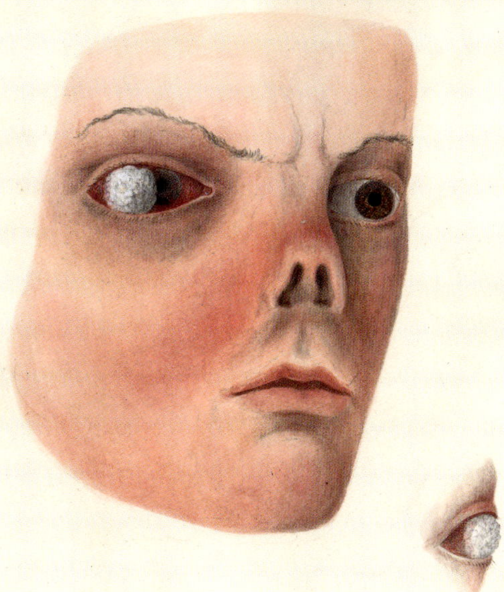

Carnucula carcinomatodes.
Protocollirt im Jahre 18$\frac{32}{33}$ No 8.

Jos. Zehner. ad. nat. del.

Fig. 77
By Gartner 1845?

Here, my first guess would be cellulitis/erysipelas of the face. A fixed "drug" eruption (perhaps a herbal toxin?) could be a differential diagnosis. I exclude acute Lupus erythematosus and dermatomyositis because of the unilateral distribution. An eczematous process can also be ruled out as I see no sign of epidermal involvement.

XI. 2. C.

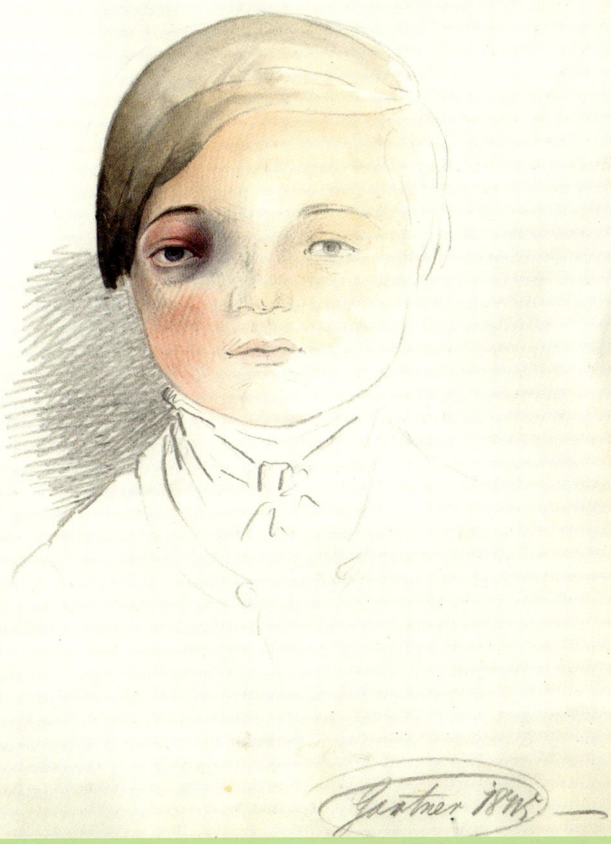

Description by Helmut Denk, pathologist

(We cannot explain the origin of this picture and why an animal brain entered the collection of ophthalmic drawings and paintings. Once included, we did not want to discard it, especially since it was by Beer's hand. So we asked a real pathologist to give us an idea of what he thought. Remark of the principal authors.)

Fig. 78
By Georg Joseph Beer

Side view (Fig. 1) and top view (Fig. 2) of the head of a duck. In Fig. 2 the skull is opened and the eyes, the eye muscles, the optic nerves and the brain are visible. The surface of the brain is rather smooth. Visible are also meningeal vessels.

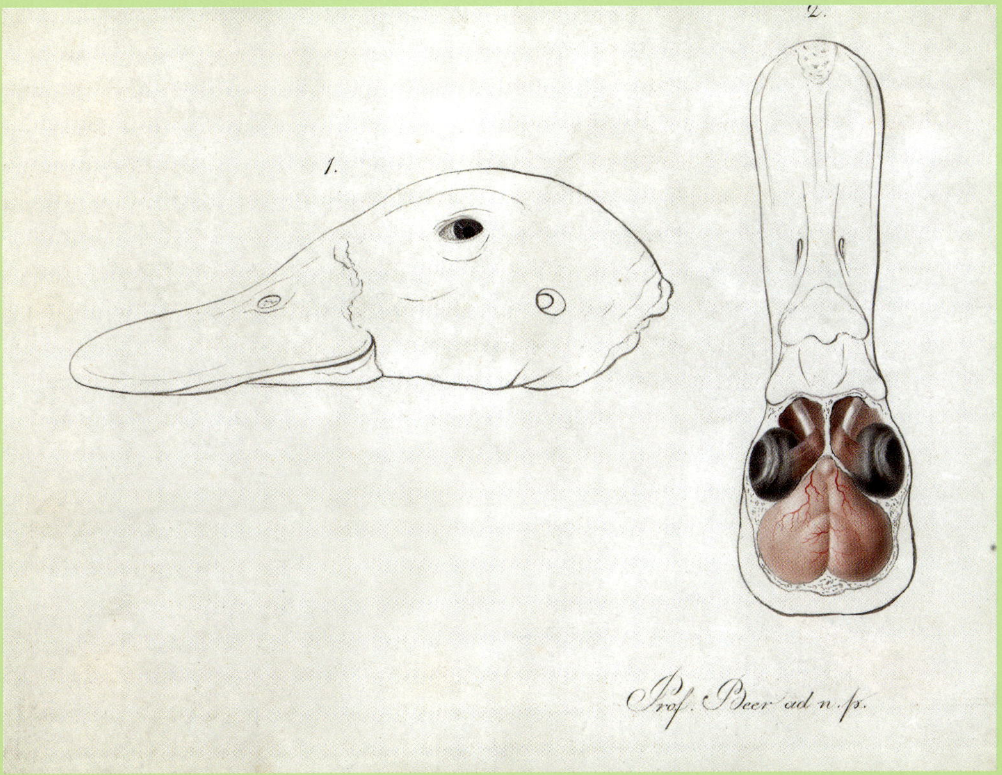
1.
2.
Prof. Beer ad n. p.

The Changing Face of Medical Terminology

DARRELL WILKINSON, dermatologist

"For the language of medicine is a verbal picture which illustrates the ideas concerning disease which civilized man has entertained over the last 2,500 years" (Roberts F.)

"Language is but the outward and visible sign of which thought is the inward and spiritual faculty" (Singer L.)

"The written word is a tricky and recalcitrant medium" (Dirckx J. H.)

"When I use a word" Humpty Dumpty said, in rather a scornful tone, "it means just what I chose it to mean - neither more nor less"
(Caroll L., Through the Looking Glass and What Alice Found)

All terminology is infinitely complex and that of technology particularly so. The language of medicine is derived both from its art and its science. Part of its art lies in communication with patients, requiring a knowledge of vernacular or common words, as well as professional terms, which comprise their "learned language". Its science evolves so rapidly that new words or new interpretation of old ones are added constantly to its terminology. Our concern here is therefore both with the changes in the meaning or concepts of old terms and with the accumulation of new ones.

Medicine in some form has been practised from the earliest times in every culture but superstition, animism or a close connection with religious beliefs dominated its art, which was usually carried out by priests or magi - the learned men of the day. Western medicine evolved from Egypt, Babylon and Assyria, where, from about 4,000 - 2,000 B.C. a quite sophisticated art and even science of medicine gradually evolved and was gradually transferred to the Aegean, starting with the Minoans and, culminating in the cult of Asclepios (Aesculapius), the "son of Apollo", whose holistic approach was allied to the treatment appropriate for the times and who created the famous "temples of healing". His daughters, Hygiea and Panacea persist as perhaps the earliest example of medical terminology, though with some modification of meaning.

From 700-300 B.C. medicine "entered a new era with the emergence of philosophers and physicians in Greece and the Aegean imbued with a spirit of inquiry about the nature of man". Plato, Pythagoras, Empedocles and Aristotle - to whom the concept of the "four humours" is attributed; and, above all, Hippocrates of Cos, born about 460 B.C. His close and repeated observation of the patient, his case-notes and continuing monitoring of signs and symptoms were allied to a rare degree of uprightness and discretion. Often called "the father of medicine", he was, in his day, the perfect physician. His theory of the balance of the "four qualities" as the foundation of health, and his copious writings on many aspects of medicine (including

"Epidemics" and the "Sacred Disease" – epilepsy) are included, together with his famous Aphorisms, in the Hippocratic collection of writings, his own and those of his followers. With the conquest of Greece by Rome, many Greek physicians went to Rome to practise, as the Romans had little interest in medicine, except as ancillaries to their armies (though their technological skills greatly improved sanitation and the quality of water). The Greek tradition persisted however, in several centres, especially Alexandria. Celsus wrote in his great work "Artes", in Latin, "De medicina" in about 30 A.D. though he made much use of Greek sources. He was greatly overshadowed, however, by Galen of Pergamon, 2nd century A.D. who wrote in Greek. He advanced the Hippocratic tradition and stressed the "body-mind" relationship. Regarded as the "father of experimental physiology" his influence was so great that he is said – somewhat unfairly – to have stultified all progress for the next 1,200 years.

The fall of Rome in 476 A.D. snuffed out medicine in Western Europe though the early writings were preserved in some monasteries and were taken over by the Arabic writers such as Rhazes and Avicenna, as Islam spread across North Africa into Spain from the 8th - 15th centuries. With the gradual re-emergence of a spirit of enquiry in the late Middle Ages, these were translated back into Latin. Each of these transcriptions involved, inevitably, errors of translation.

This resurgence burst into flame at the Renaissance, particularly in Italy and, though more tardily, in countries across the Alps. In this intense re-awakening of intellectual curiosity arose figures such as Leonardo, Vesalius, Sanctorius and Fracastoro, who coined the word, "Syphilis" from the swineherd in his poem. With new modes of thought and concepts of causation, other new terms appeared and increased continually in the subsequent ages of discovery and innovation. For the most part these were described in Graeco-Latin formations, sometimes hybrid, sometimes corrupted, even when the knowledge of Greek was in decline though Latin continued to be used for most medical textbooks until the 18th century.

The invention of printing in the 15th century revolutionised the spread of knowledge and made it available in all countries, where medical terms were often codified in the vernacular or regional language. The practical use of the microscope by van Leeuwenhoek of Holland (1632–1723), Auenbrugger's (1722–1809) percussion method of 1761, Laennec's stethoscope of 1819 and von Helmholtz' ophthalmoscope in 1851 enabled hitherto dark corners to be explored. In the 17th century Harvey discovered the circulation of the blood and Sydenham, the "English Hippocrates", gave clear accounts of malaria, plague, smallpox and hysteria and defined gout and cholera. His insistence on observation rather than theory laid the foundation of modern medicine. Hunter (1728–1793) combined anatomy with pathology and James Lind in his treatise on "Scurvy" in 1753 advocated fresh fruit or lime juice, eliminating their cause of considerable incapacity at sea. Lady Wortley Montague (1689–1762), then in Constantinople, practised inoculating with smallpox but it was Edward Jenner (1749–1823) who substituted inoculation with cowpox and began the eradication of this fearsome disease.

The age of modern medicine was ushered in by many other famous names - Boerhaave, Claude Bernard, Charcot, Virchow, Pasteur, Semmelweis, Koch, Lister and many others, each famous in his own way and each adding some new term or interpretation of disease. More recently, the discovery of x-rays, of penicillin and subsequent antibiotics, of cortisone and its derivates, of retinoids, immuno-modulators, the unravelling of DNA and the birth of immunochemistry have led to new languages of their own and the current attempts at cloning and stem-cell research will doubtless add to these.

Forms of Language

Terminology varies considerably with different forms of language and expression. We have mentioned Professional and Vernacular forms. One should add variations of these such as Argot, peculiar to a particular trade, society or profession and not always understood by the "uninitiated"; Dialect, differing from region to region within one country; Slang, informal (and often private) vernacular; and Jargon, a form of chatter sometimes used as a synonym for Argot, i.e., "medical jargon". All these play a part in the terminology of disease, in whatever language it is expressed.

Though Greek stems remain faithful to their classical roots, Latin evolved into Late Latin and then Italian and, with Provencal, formed the basis for the Romance languages. The Teutonic tongues Frankish and Burgundian had their own variations, the Southern dialect forming modern German and Austrian, the Northern and Western (Plattdeutsch) becoming Dutch and Flemish and Old Norse forming the basis of the Scandinavian tongues.
English, with its multiple roots, reached its apogee in the 16th century after reaching its cohesion in the 14th century, as in Chaucer. Description of diseases has been expressed vibrantly by Shakespeare, though the first great English dictionary, by Johnson, did not appear until 1755. The richness of its vocabulary has led to its predominance as the international language of medicine in place of Latin. The Slavic countries tended for long to preserve their own terms and Greece will allow only Greek roots.

Forms of Change and Development

Mistranslation and transcription have already been noted. Incorporation of terms from other European countries include such words as malaria, belladonna and pellagra (Italian), pinta and cascara (Spanish) albino - ex L., albus - (Portugal) and some of the shorter Germanic words such as Kernicterus and mast cell ("stuffed").

With the opening of trade routes and exploration, new terms were introduced from distant countries; yaws, kwashiorkor (red boy), beri-beri, etc. In more recent times American English has exerted an appreciable effect, increasingly introduced, with its transposition or elision of letters such as "er" for "re", of "u" in honour, tumour, etc., the deletion of ligatures and the suppression of the final "al" as in physiologic.

Contraction, a change from the general to the particular is shown by "eclampsia", used by Hippocrates for any illness occurring like a flash of light (Gr., lampas) and typhus (from Gr., typhos, smoke, mist) originally described the stupor of those in fever. "Morbus", L., disease, giving rise to morbilli, measles. In Expansion the meaning of a term was extended. Nausea was originally only sea-sickness and epithelium was originally applied to the skin over the nipple (Gr., thele). Corruption is common, especially in vernacular terms, e.g., "shingles" from cingulum, L., belt, "plague" from plege, Gr., a blow, "goitre" from L., guttus, throat and so on. In the 14th century the Beth-le-hem hospital for the insane was corrupted to "Bedlam", now itself extinct, and an example of Euphemism, the change from offensive to more polite terms. Aphesis, the loss of an initial letter, is seen in "squint", originally M.E. asquint.

Reversal of meaning is less common but shown, for example, in "phlegmatic" originally the opposite as Gr., phlegein to burn; and "L., valgus", originally bow-legged.

Transfer of one meaning or concept to another is common and often seen in the 17th–18th centuries. Galen used "atheroma" for a tumour containing a gruel-like substance such as a sebaceous cyst but is now applied to lumpy deposits in arteries; rheumatism arose from O.E., "rheum", Gr., rheo, to flow, a discharge from nose or eyes, transferred to the flowing of the "humour" in old parlance the cause of rheumatism. Hysteria (from Gr., hyster, womb) and hypochondria (from the concept of melancholy deriving from the liver and spleen) are self-evident. Focus, L., was originally a fire in the centre of the room, now the central point of attention or discussion and - more obliquely - graft originally arises from the Gr., graphein, to write, derived from the pencil-like pointed stems used for grafting trees.

On the other hand, some Graeco-Latin terms or their Romance derivatives have persisted, though their cause or formation has changed, e.g., "acromegaly" for a state of large ends", pellagra, from rough skin and granuloma. Malaria - bad air - existed long before the mosquito entered the picture and "herpes" was originally any spreading eruption.

Some terms are of confused or unknown origin. Thymus, Gr., thymos, heart, (also the plant thyme), was used for any wartlike excrescence akin to the plant's flowers and also to the gland in the chest of young animals. Cretin, now obsolete as derogatory is said to be derived from an offensive word for early Christians. Astragalus had eight different meanings - the upper cervical vertebra (Homer), the talus (Hippocrates) etc., perhaps, as Roberts suggests, because tale, dice, were used for any form of dice-gambling.

Prefixes and Suffixes modify the root or give meaning to the use of a term. They are mostly well-known. Though chiefly Greek in origin, there are some exceptions such as "unci-" L., twisted, as in uncineria, "per" L., thorough(ly), as in pertussis; and "mis-" (O.E., wrong) or "mid-". Some less common or newly introduced ones include:

en-, em-, in, among, as in epidemics, ana – throughout, led to "anasarca" now obsolete for oedema. dia – through, both in a general sense and as diascopy (Unna) coined for seeing into the skin by pressure of glass. ide (or -id in modern English) for a skin condition associated with but distant to the original disease; tuberculid, trichophytid.

- centesis. Puncturing a cavity to aspirate fluid
- ase for forms of enzymes
- ia, state of, like. In French is -ie and in English -y

Sometimes adjectival terms are used as in pellagra It. ex L., rough skin and podagra, from Gr., pous, podos, foot and agra, pain, for gout in moderate terms.

Synonyms, the use of different names for the same disease according to national differences or vernacular usage. Thus, brucellosis (named after Sir David Bruce) is also called undulant, Malta, goat fever, etc. They are sometimes a useful form of shorthand in professional speech.

Eponyms are much more common and still widely used throughout Europe and particularly so in dermatology and ophthalmology. Named after the discoverer (or sometimes the patient as in "Mortimer's Malady" – sarcoidosis), they are in both professional and vernacular use, though chiefly the former. Some examples are Alzheimer's disease, Addison's disease, Pott's fracture, Raynaud's disease and phenomenon. Cheyne-Stokes breathing and Fallot's tetralogy are confined to professional use. A few eponyms are named after places where they were first discovered or are particularly prevalent, e.g., Lyme disease (borreliosis) from the original cases in a town in Massachusets, Mal de Meleda after an Adriatic island and "Delhi boil or Aleppo boil" for Leishmaniasis. Alone, the Rhesus factor is named after a type of monkey. A very few have become words in their own right, e.g., pasteurisation.

There are some oddities and some deceptions. Among the former, Galen, is perpetuated only in the obsolescent term "galenicals". Sadism, masochism and narcissism have kept the name of their mentors but lost their capital initials. "Sister Joseph's nodule" is named after a Sister at the Mayo clinic, who observed its significance. The colourful "St. Vitus" dance and "St. Anthony's fire" are, alas, no longer with us. The deceptions arise in various forms. "Grenz rays" are due, not to a person but to the German capitalisation of nouns, grenz meaning "margin". Grave's disease in English is Basedow's in German and so on. Two diseases may have the same eponym, e.g., Paget's disease of the nipple and of the bone (osteitis deformans). And two or more authors may describe the same disease, when it becomes cumbersome as in the Fiessinger-Le Roy syndrome (Reiter's disease); or two different diseases as in the Goltz-Gorlin and the Gorlin-Goltz syndromes.

Acronyms are a form of verbal shorthand, abundant in medicine and unfortunately gaining credence in common parlance. Some are acceptable as they help in doctor-patient communication – VD, ENT, HIV etc. AIDS, one of the most recent, is now firmly established but is known differently in different countries, becoming SIDA in France and SPID in Russia. Acronyms are particularly common in the immunological field, where they form a private professional argot but their widespread growth in medicine should, I feel, be resisted.

Finally, the demands of euphony often override strict accuracy of words, such as the derivation from the genitive of the stem. And custom and usage – "jus et norma loquendi" (Horace) – regulate all forms of language. Medicine is no exception.

In this summary of the complexities of medical terminology it is not possible to include many of the numerous examples of the types of change that have been outlined. But a few of interest include:
ranula, from Gr., rana, frog. Retentive cyst of salivary gland, used by Virgil for a swelling of the tongue in some animals.

scrofula, dim. of scrofa, L., a sow, from the resemblance of swollen glands of the neck to that of a pig.

tragus, from L., goat, Gr., tragos. For that part of the ear that has tufts of hair like a goat's chin.

botulism, from botulus, sausage, from original cases from contaminated sausages.

porphyria, from porphyreos Gr., purple, from the colour of the urine in attacks.

cheloid, from chele Gr., claw. From its resemblance to a crayfish's claws. But Addison later confused the issue with his "keloid" from kele, Gr., a scar. But this incorrect spelling for the tumour unfortunately persists.

chorea, Gr., dance. For the involuntary movements in Huntington's and Sydenham's diseases.

diabetes, Gr., used until 16th century for polyuria, then, with mellitus added, as "honeyed passing through".

hormone, Gr., hormao an assault, to set in motion or arouse.

hypnosis, Gr., hypnosso to fall asleep. Braid (1796–1860) introduced "hypnotism". But now known to differ from sleep.

Some terms that have changed their meaning include:
psora, Gr., scab, itch. Now as in psoriasis, a non-itching disease. lupus, L., wolf. Used as lupus vulgaris for the eroding lesion of tuberculosis and, less aptly, for lupus erythematosus. anastomosis, Gr. Galen used it as an "opening-up", now, a joining together. autopsy, Gr. properly, "self-seeing". Hardly apt.

In the present context it is appropriate to include some ophthalmological terms. Like dermatology, it is a particularly visual specialty and many old terms are derived from natural objects or patterns and have remained unchanged: lens, from its lentil-like shape, cornea from L., corneus, horny, sclera from the Gr., scleros hard, dacryon, Gr., a tear, hordoleum, L., barleycorn, from the shape and size and pterygium from Gr., pteryx a little wing, an apt term for the vascular growth of the conjunctiva spreading from the edge to the centre; and others.

Somewhat more oblique in origin are: iris, from Gr., rainbow or colourful aura encircling a central area; pupil, from L., pupilla, dim. of pupa, doll, the resemblance of oneself in another's eye; and chalazion of Gr., chalax, hailstone, used by Galen for a pimple on the eyelid.

Of particular interest are:
cataract, from Gr., kataraktes, L., cataracta. Both a waterfall and a sluice-gate or portcullis, to control the flow.

glaucoma, originally from glaux, Gr., owl. Homer's epithet for Athena was glaukopis, owl-faced, as depicted on Greek coins. "Glaukos" means both gleaming and a bluish-green colour. Victorian translators gave it as "grey-eyed Athena".

glaucoma, as a neuter noun was used by Hippocrates as a form of cataract and, glaucosis as "blindness" from glaucoma.

A great many descriptive terms have changed in meaning or their causes have become clarified, especially since the discovery of the ophthalmoscope by von Helmholtz in 1851 and the introduction and development of the microscope:

keratoconjunctivitis is now divided into at least fifteen different varieties.
trachoma, originally a "roughness" of the conjunctiva is now known to be due to Chlamydia infection.

hypopyon from Gr., hypopyos, "tending to suppurate" (Hippocrates) is now confined to suppuration of the anterior chamber.

staphyloma, Gr., staphyle, grape. Now applies to a bulge at the back of the sclera, causing myopia.

coloboma, Gr., kolobos, shortened, docked, is extended to encompass not only congenital defects of the eyelids but also notching of lens, iris or retina.

melanosis bulbi oculi is now defined in several different causes.
pladaroma, from Gr., plados, moist, soft, pladao, to be flaccid. Hippocrates used "plada-

ros" as a state of moistness. The term itself is first attributed to the lexicographer Suidas. Best translated as "pliable".

Terms for distortions or defects of vision often remain unchanged, such as presbyopia and astigmatism, though some have also changed their meaning to some degree:

myopia, from Gr., myops, -opis, to close eyes, blink, thus for short-sightedness. nystagmus, from Gr., nystazein to nod or sleep. Originally drowsiness as of nodding of head, then to sporadic oscillatory movements of the eyes.

nyctalopia, paradoxical, with a dual meaning, from Gr., nyx, night, alaos, blind and ops, eye, as "tes nyctos alaos" (Galen). The common meaning accepted in English is "night-blindness", or defective "dark adaptation", as in a dim light or after sunset. But Galen also adds the contrary; "ability to see better at night" as with some mammals and birds and, rarely, in man. Both definitions given in OED, though the latter considered "erroneous". It is, however, used in this way in several continental countries – "faculté de voir pendant le nuit ou l'obscurité". Originally by Hippocrates as "seeing better in a dim light" and by Galen as "blind by night" but later, erroneously by loss of "alaos" as seeing better by night. Now used in English for "night-blindness" and in French as "day-blindness".

Many new terms have thus evolved from a better definition of old ones such as chorioiditis and retinitis with the increasing use of refinements in technical advances, the development of histology and advances in knowledge of general medical conditions with ophthalmic involvement, such as diabetes, sarcoidosis, ulcerative colitis, pseudoxanthoma elasticum and a host of syndromes and varieties of infection, most recently Lyme disease and AIDS.

New surgical techniques have long since overtaken the simple "couching" for cataracts practised over 2000 years ago and the advent of laser and plastic surgery has produced its own specialised terminology.

This explosion of scientific technology, microbiology, biochemistry and genotype unravelling in the past hundred years has led to a far greater understanding of the causes and implications of diseases of the eye and their investigation, treatment and prevention. The present concern is to bring these advances in Western Medicine to the rest of the world.

Acknowledgements

I am greatly indebted to several colleagues for their comments and suggestions and to Colin Badcock, for his unfailing help.
The subject has been extensively studied by many authors. I have gained in particular from:
Dirckx JH: The Language of Medicine. 2nd ed. Praeger, New York, 1983
Kanski JJ: Clinical Ophthalmology. 4th ed. Butterworth Heinemann, Oxford, 1999
Roberts F. Medical Terms. London, Heinemann, 1954

Vision and Fiction:
The Eye and Visual Perception as a Metaphor in Literature

Marita Amm, ophthalmologist

"Open then, mine eyes, your double sluice ...
Thus let your streams o'erflow your springs,
Till eyes and tears be the same things:
And each the other's difference bears;
These weeping eyes, those seeing tears."
Andrew Marvell, Eyes and Tears, Complete poems

Theories dealing with the hierarchy of the senses lead to different results at different times. The question whether this change of mind (change of the senses) has its source in social conventions and subjectivism, whether sensory physiology is continuously developing with different weight and influence of environment, or whether the hierarchy of the senses is a historically constant, determined by the genes and early evolution, - this question remains a work for the social and cultural sciences. In literature the eye stays privileged over the other four senses.

In all ages and in all regions writers considered the eye, this outpost of the brain, to have a special influence and power. Eyesight played a critical role in shaping a human's perspective and communication. "Sight integrates the other senses" postulated John Hull, the blind professor of theology and philosophy in Birmingham, the way we respond to and reflect on our world is strongly associated with our eyesight. So a rich ocular symbolization and codification in prose, poetry, philosophy and prophecy developed and offer evidence to the exposed position of this organ in our sensuous experience and appreciation(1).

We can distinguish two main groups in the variety of eye metaphors and in the long list of visual terms, visual idioms, stylistic devices and symbols, revealing an important visual basis to the categories of abstraction and attraction:

The seeing eye and
The blind eye.

The seeing eye

Passive and active role of the outer eye
The lyric eye: aesthetics and aura
The magic eye: characterization of internal nature and creation of external atmosphere

The active role of the inner, the mind's or the third eye
The eye and I: personality determining feature
The overseeing and foreseeing eye: "voir = savoir"

The mighty and the thinking eye
The evil eye
The instrument of the nonverbal communication and the erotic eye. The eye as a witness
Vice versa: the eye as a producer of illusion

The blind eye

Punishment
Seeing with "other eyes"
Freedom from the domination of visual stimuli
Resistance against revelation
Synonym for repression

Passive and active role of the outer eye

Mostly the writers describe and admire the attraction by the beauty of the outer eye. Its individual variations and its sparkling, charming color have inspired poets to exuberant hymns: The love poems of Sappho, Ovidius or Heinrich Heine, the Roman de la rose [1234] by Guillaume de Lorris, the tale Ligeia by Edgar Allen Poe. The aestetics and aura, the loveliness and expression of this organ of sense are directly correlated with the inter-

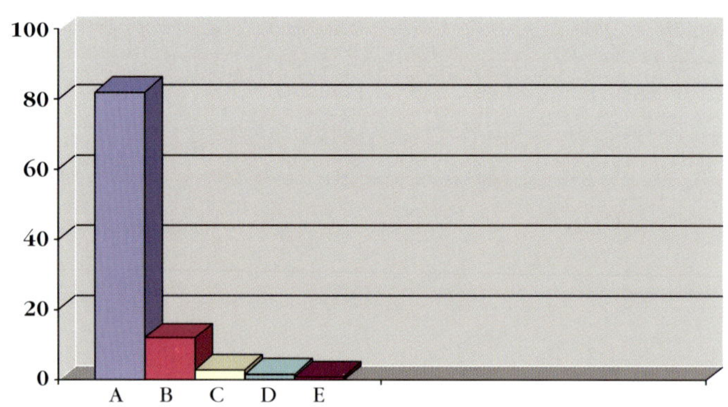

Fig. 79

Hierarchy of the senses: A - seeing, B - hearing, C - sense of smell, D - sense of touch, E - sense of taste (Wulf Winkeloos: Architektur und Raum, Sehen und Sichtbarmachen, Stuttgart 1985).

nal and individual character and moral excellence of the hero. But not only the beauty and perfection of the eye imply a reflection of heart and soul. Also the defective eye, especially the squinting eye transfers a message, mostly the information of a bad character and despicableness. A heterogeneous, but generally terrifying and disastrous representation is connected with the eye of the Cyclopes (Kyklopia = the country of the eyes is the name for a region near Naples with the opikoi, the people of the eyes).

The magic of the eyes: The eye is attractive and alarming. It induces a permanent oscillation between veracity and virtual reality, fact and fiction. The transparency of the cornea and lens gives an impression of candour, which is perhaps synonymous with a feeling of trustworthiness and truthfulness. But the pupil is also a deep, dark, impenetrable hole, a quasi-mystical aperture. The incessant movement of the eyes and their morphologies as used by authors like E. A. Poe, Mary Shelley and many representatives of the "Gothic novel", create a mysterious, transcendent atmosphere in their novels. The same intention can be found in German Romanticism (Ludwig Tieck: The Runic Mountain; Joseph von Eichendorff: The Marmor Statue).

The active role of the inner, the mind's or the third eye

The extraordinary anatomy of the eye predestines it to be a personality determining feature. The so created absolute autonomy of this organ does not require a body, acts sovereignly. This connotation is effectively expressed by the nightmare about the eye of conscience (Dostoyevski's Crime and Punishment and J. J. Grandville's First Dream, Criminal and Penance). The eye is equivalent to the person and sufficient to identify a subject. There is an interesting reference to the high status of the eye as identity forming energy in the English title of the novel Soglyadatay by Vladimir Nabokov: The Eye. Eye is homophonous with I. The thus defined congruence intensifies the basic message of the text: incessant self-observation as an individual attempt to save an existence that has lost its own center.

In Christianity the (all-seeing) eye represents God. In the same meaning of omnipotence and omniscience, but also as a protective device, the motif was adopted for the Great Seal of the United States of America (to be seen on the one Dollar bill). In ancient Egypt the eye was the symbol of the god Horus and a hieroglyphic standing for the hope for salvation and rebirth of mankind.

The anatomical conditions of the eye, which allow a direct contact between the world without and the world within (the optic nerve is the only visible cerebral structure, and as such it can be directly examined), make it an instrument that can transcend the mere physical process of looking. It becomes a tool for overseeing, foreseeing, recognizing and associating. In antiquity and literature we find the synonym eye and sun, (eye-)light and life. In Timaeus, Plato saw visual perception as having a key position among the senses. He stressed the related nature of eye (phosphora ommata), light and sun, putting vision into a religious-philosophical context. And centuries later in their discourses on light, enlightenment and elucidation, the intellectuals and scientists of the 17th and 18th century devoted themselves to investigating the epistemological aspects of perception. The eye took on a metaphysical status; seeing was a holistic process. Goethe wrote: "Sight is the noblest sense: the other four inform us via our organs of tactile apprehension: we hear, feel, smell, touch by contact; sight, however, is of infinitely higher standing, rises more subtly above what is material and gets close to spiritual faculties" (Maxims and Reflections).

The evolutionary affinity of eyes and brain suggests a functional, emotional and cognitive affinity between the two[(5)]. Perception is a highly interlinked process, starting at the retina with the endpoint of the brain as its computing neural system. Seeing assumes the status of a requirement for thinking (in renaissance and later in enlightenment), the more, the eye in literature is used as a synonym for the work done by the brain in processing and filtering impressions. The resolution and acuity of the optic system determine the resolution and the acuity of the mind. Beside the intellectual capability the eye takes over a psychoanalytical function. With the figurative and active functions of a reflective, diagnostic or commentating view writers discover an inward turning vision, a self-reflection and the chance to gain deeper insights, e.g., Cees Nooteboom – Het gezicht van het oog, the Austrian Christoph Ransmayr – Morbus Kitahara. The title employs the poetic sounding name for chorioretinopathia centralis serosa. This component of the eye exemplifies an independent, intellectual authority, the responsible human being.

All cultures know the concept of the evil eye and its destructive potential. Its powerful influence emanates primarily from the pathologically altered eye and symbolizes corruption, morbidity, diseases and death. Many manifestations of the evil eye are found in fairytales, legends and myths and in rabbinic literature: Griaule M. – Œil, mauvais œil. According to the Talmud, the Angel of Death is perceived as having eyes everywhere, meaning according to one interpretation that nothing can escape him and the dying cannot avoid his stare[(6)]. The eye is one of the most expressive organs of nonverbal communication, an eloquent gauge of our feelings and emotions. We regard the unmistakable expression of the eyes as a more reliable communicator than any mutable word. It is not only the eye of Eros as in the title of a painting by Paul Klee, 1919, but, conversely, the Eros of the eye that caresses, bewitches, seduces. A glance from eye to eye is the elemental, existential sine qua non at all levels of interpersonal contacts, e.g., William Shakespeare: Romeo and Juliet, The Winter's tale; Joseph Turnley: The language of the eye; James Joyce: Ulysses; Jean Starobinsky: The living eye. The power of love and eros starts with the glance, often at first glance. In Ulysses each of the 18 episodes represents an organ. The 13th episode, Nausikaa, the flirt – the giving the eye – between Leopold Bloom and Gerty MacDowell, has as its underlying organ the eye. The eye became the medium through which sensuality and sensitivity were perceived and expressed. An injury to such a sensitive tissue hurts also emotionally, is a provocation, as described by Georges Bataille in L'Histoire de l' œil[(2)].

The development of imagery and speech are closely linked to the functional capacity of our eyesight. We trust primarily the reality and veracity conveyed to us by our eyes. This is the basis of much of our initial experience of the world and our orientation; on it we erect our language and our writing systems. Testimony by an eyewitness is considered to be more trustworthy than hearsay evidence. "What we learn only through the ears impresses less upon our minds than what is presented to the trustworthy eye" (Horace).

The eye is not only regarded as a transmitter of what is authentic and accurate, confident and certain, but equally as a producer of illusions. It is endowed with a capacity for projective perception. Thus the metaphor eye can lead us to a different level, that of vision and imagination, to a creative modulation of perception. With the help of the ocular motif authors have reflected on how manipulable the senses are, how easily deceived: Edgar Allan Poe; The Spectacles; Ernst Theodor Amadeus Hoffmann: The Sandman; Ingeborg Bachmann: You happy Eyes. The confusion of the eye due to the inundation of images leads to a confusion of the brain, a frequent topic of modern authors (Michel Houllebecq, Arnold Stadler).

The blind eye

The apotheosis of independence, autonomy and sovereignity is seen as being closely connected with the intactness of the eye. Blindness signifies mostly a strict punishment (Oedipus, Hecuba and Polymestor). But the reception of blindness is different in different cultures. In the Christian culture blindness is often seen under the aspect of moral standards, in an aura of sin, infidelity and death, parallel with intellectual blindness (transcendental blindness) (José Saramago: Ensayo sobre la ceguera).

As a counterpart to this negative iconography and "occidental ocular tyranny"[(4)] blindness is positively connotated in most of the oriental societies and cultures. It is interpreted as a chance for intensified perception. This philosophical dimension traces an undistracted vision that develops out of itself, that dissociates itself from the all too easily deluded and seduced eyesight. It symbolizes serenity, internal equilibrium and foresight, e.g., Teiresias, the blind seer of ancient mythology; Christa Wolff: Cassandra; Hervé Guibert: Des aveugles.

But he, though blind of sight,
despised and thought extinguished quite,
with inward eyes illuminated,
his fiery virtue roused
from under ashes into sudden flame.

Samson Agonistes by John Milton (suffering himself from glaucoma, resulting in blindness 1652). Blindness – a world where perceptions of sound, silence and space are greatly changed – offers a chance to escape the pure physiology of optic occupation.

The loss of the visual acuity and the loss of optical control allow a seeing with other eyes and open the experience of independence from visual stimuli. Blindness gives a liberation from the obsession of a visual-voyeuristic control, a new definition of a "memory space" (Elias Canetti: "Blinding - Die Blendung").

This form of freedom from the dictatorship of the eyes means also a protection from the superabundance and simultaneousness of signs, signals and stimuli, which attack the eyes in the modern media world with an almost obsessive frenzy of image making, forming more and more bizarre impressions.

Other interpretations of (hysteric, psychologically determined) blindness are a resistance against revelation (Ernst Weiss: The Eyewitness; Marguerite Duras: Hiroshima, mon amour) and a synonym for repression (Sigmund Freud).

Conclusion

Since the renaissance, until the beginning of the 20th century the hierarchy of the senses was characterized by a dominance of the visual sense. Especially in literature the eye played the dominant aesthetic position in aesthesis, the sensual presence and perception. It functioned as a main stylistic device to identify an inner and outer personality. Beyond the descriptive element the eye served as a condition for abstract thoughts. Abstract thinking is linked to the visual system. Perception provides the foundation for apperception. The thinking is seeing formula of Marcel Danesi (and reversible equation) represents the extraordinary significance, charisma and energy connected with the eye in literature and speech[(3)].

Simultaneously, scepticism against the eye as the prime sense and sole guarantee for objectivity was already discussed in the 13th century (William of Ockham). A rebellion against the predominance of the eye and a request for reform arose. Later Johann Gottfried Herder postulated the tactile sense as the most important human sense, Diderot located the soul in our skin[(4)]. But in the written lyrics, the eye remained the most adored organ.

Modern and post-modern literature and philosophy increasingly opposes this monocular conception. There is a deconstruct of authority and absolutism of the eye and visual objectivity is called into question. Authors like Franz Kafka and Ingeborg Bachmann warned of the inundation of the images and the inflation of visual objects with the risk of an uniformed eye and demand an interplay of the senses with the intention of a feeling and touching eye and a seeing hand.

The new definition of a harmony of the sensual system may be seen in the regained interest in Johann Gottfried Herder, who criticized the scoptophily and rehabilitated the haptic sense as a central sense for comprehending reality[(7)]. The Nobel Prize in medicine

2004 for the research into the sense of smell to Linda B. Buck and Richard Axel, and the return of the theories of the French physician Alfred Tomatis, who postulated and promoted the ear and aural sense as the most important sense for the human being, point in this direction.

A plurality and a renewed contemplation of a more balanced pentagon of the senses appear necessary to fix the position of mankind in the world.

It is only with the heart that one can see rightly; what is essential is invisible to the eye Antoine de Saint Exupery.

References

(1) Amm M: Might and magic, lust and language – the eye as a metaphor in literature. Documenta Ophthalmologica 101: 223–232; 2000

(2) Barthes R: Die Augenmetapher. In: Helga Galles (ed). Strukturalismus als interpretatives Verfahren. Luchterhand, Darmstadt 1972

(3) Danesi M: Thinking is seeing: Visual metaphors and the nature of abstract thought. Semiotica 1990; 80: 221–237

(4) Derrida J: Mémoires d'aveugle. L'autoportrait et autres ruines. Editions de la Réunion des musées nationaux. 1990

(5) Gregory RL: Origin of eyes and brains. Nature 1967; 213:369–372

(6) Kemp W: Sehsucht: Die Engführung. In: Kunst- und Ausstellungshalle der Bundesrepublik Deutschland (Pontus Hulten) (eds). Sehsucht. Schriftenreihe Forum. Steidl, Göttingen 1995: 53–66

(7) Zeuch U: Umkehr der Sinneshierarchie. Herder und die Aufwertung des Tastsinnes seit der frühen Neuzeit, Niemeyer, Tübingen 2000

tively, the interaction of memory and imagination may activate sensory cortices and, as a result, affect the activities of frontal or motor cortices as well. Furthermore, a change of motivation or affect may modulate the flow of information from posterior to frontal cortices. These factors control the perception-action cycle and are inseparable with regard to their effects. This has several important implications. First, the distinction of objective and subjective qualities of experience looses its significance. Second, an indefinite number of new structures of perception and action may be generated within the perception-action cycle thus giving rise to what has been termed creative intelligence. Third, the quality of integration embodied in the perception-action cycle makes Gestalt phenomenology a particularly useful paradigm for the study of brain and aesthetics.

Beauty as the impact of Gestalt

In 1890 Baron Christian von Ehrenfels, the founder of Gestalt psychology, wrote: "The impact of Gestalt (German: Höhe der Gestalt) increases with the product of its components, its organisation, and the manifold of its parts. The whole of aesthetics may be based on Gestalt theory if the concept of the impact of Gestalt is taken into account. What we term Beauty is nothing else than the impact of Gestalt. A low impact of Gestalt means ugliness." Other authors of the time expressed similar ideas. The Harvard mathematician George D. Birkhoff (1933) sought to cast them into the mould of a quantitative relation. He contended that the aesthetic measure of a work of art, M, is the product of two factors, namely its degree of order (O) and the inverse (1/C) of its structural complexity, that is, $M = O/C$. Birkhoff verified this relation for a large number of examples of geometric figures, lines of poetry, and music. Further studies of experimental aesthetics were conducted by Eysenck (1941), who was led to replace Birkhoff's rule by the equation $M = O \cdot C$.

It appears that the inconsistency of the concepts of Birkhoff and Hans Jürgen Eysenck results from the incongruence of their categories of description. Birkhoff, very much like Abraham A. Moles (1966) and Raul Gunzenhäuser (1968) in their later approach of information aesthetics, based his aesthetic theory on physical properties of the stimulus. Eysenck, by contrast, relied on the statistical analysis of observer judgments by means of psychometric methodologies. The underlying concept of the psychological space leaves the relations between physical stimulus features, or attributes, and their mental representations largely unspecified. Such problems have been addressed by the cognitive turn of psychology. Accordingly, a given stimulus may give rise to different types of response depending on the internal state of the organism. Hence the expectation that the impact of different stimulus dimensions on the aesthetic response varies with that state. In other words, the origin of beauty is to be sought for in the brain of the observer.

On these grounds we explored the potentials of neuroaesthetics by considering the relationships of visual perception and aesthetic preference(5). We found the aesthetic preference for moderately complex patterns to be systematically related to stimulus attributes of structure, or form, but varying with object knowledge. For one class of images, termed compound Gabor patterns, we were able to demonstrate that the relationship is determined by the independent factors of complexity and symmetry. The acquisition of categorical concepts for these stimuli through learning selectively affected these factors: While the complexity factor was varied by category learning, the symmetry factor was not. These findings obviously contradict Kant, according to whom there should be no dependency whatsoever between the aesthetic judgment and knowledge.

For resolving the discrepancies of traditional aesthetics and results of cognitive research, we employed concepts from machine intelligence for analysing visual performance. Image segmentation, feature or attribute extraction, and the generation of classification rules are defined here with regard to the physical image domain. Structural information is preserved in the representational format by describing patterns, or more generally images and scenes, in terms of parts and their part-specific and part-relational attributes. We then used algorithms from machine learning to characterise perceptual categorization as a sequence of tests of working hypotheses. Each hypothesis corresponds to the selection of a subset of attributes, which defines a reference system for describing pattern structure. Once selected, the elaboration of such a hypothesis warrants the formation of rules and the tuning of evidence weights. Eventually, the elaboration process results in successful categorisation, or the current hypothesis is rejected and replaced by an alternative one. It can be said therefore that such procedures provide pattern descriptions, the validity of which is context dependent.

The resulting cognitive relativity of pattern classification has its theoretical foundation in the Theorem of the Ugly Duckling of mathematical logics[(6)]. It states that the number of predicates shared by any two objects is constant, independent of the choice of the two objects, provided that a finite set of predicates or attributes is used. These attributes need be capable of distinguishing any two objects considered. The proof of this theorem rests on the possibility to construct predicates of higher rank that are shared by these objects. The disturbing consequence of this result is that a swan and a duck, and two swans are equally similar[(7)]. This would seem to be the death-blow to any attempt of using the concept of similarity as a basis of categorisation. Yet there exists the possibility of resurrecting it by replacing in the definition of similarity the enumeration of shared predicates by the value-oriented ponderation of shared predicates. Indeed, if some predicates are treated as more "important" than others, the notion of similarity can be based on a measure that specifies the extent to which more important predicates are shared.

Embodied Aesthetics

The present considerations would seem to suggest that the value-oriented ponderation of object attributes for pattern classification and aesthetic preference are two sides of one coin. It should be noted, however, that in case of category learning novel occurrences have to be related to learned class descriptions. To allow the continuous updating of such descriptions during learning, they have to be kept in working memory or, in physiological terms, in prefrontal cortex. This would imply that the fit of input patterns to class descriptions in working memory entails the aesthetic response. Interestingly enough, however, current research in cognitive neuroscience suggests that feedback signals from the high-level visual understanding system are sent to some mesolimbic system. Thus we are led to propose that the visual aesthetic response to pattern stimuli has two major components, namely value-oriented ponderation of object attributes within some high-level visual understanding system and an emotional response from feedback between the high-level system and limbic structures in the brain.

We are then left with the question of how predicate importance for value-driven evaluation is determined. The answer is related to the biological origin of human values. Within the span of two million years, when evolution shaped the brain of homo sapiens, he/she was mainly concerned with issues of life and death. Is this a branch, which may be used as a weapon, or is it a poisonous serpent? Can this be eaten or will it devour me? The ability of the brain to decide about such crucial matters in an instance enabled humans to survive. It can be said therefore that the biological origin of human values is the need to evaluate sensory experience with regard to decisions concerning life and death. Only if these decisions were well-taken, was there a chance to arrive at socially relevant decisions and, finally, to endeavour the cultural refinement of values.

The view of human intelligence being shaped by what is most important for survival warrants the conclusion that it is not adequately characterised by solely focusing on logic and reasoning in artificial situations. This insight has led to new developments in Artificial Intelligence resulting in the concept of Embodied Intelligence. Here we argued that human aesthetics is not sufficiently characterised by the theory of the good and the true. Instead we suggested that the visual aesthetic response consists of the combined effects of value-oriented attribute evaluation for pattern categorisation within working memory and emotional activation caused by feedback signals to limbic structures. Thus, it seems that the concept of Embodied Intelligence should be complemented by the concept of Embodied Aesthetics based on the impact of Gestalt.

References

(1) Faas E: The Genealogy of Aesthetics. Cambridge University Press, Cambridge 2002

(2) Rentschler I, Epstein D, Herzberger B, eds: Beauty and the Brain. Biological Aspects of Aesthetics. Birkhäuser, Basel 1988. (Japanese Translation: Bio No Kara Kangaeru. Shinyosha Publishers, Tokyo 2000)

(3) Edelman GM: Neural Darwinism. The Theory of Neuronal Group Selection. Basic Books, New York 1987

(4) Fuster JM: Cortex and Mind. Oxford University Press, Oxford 2003

(5) Rentschler I, Jüttner M, Unzicker A, Landis T: Innate and learned components of human visual preference. Current Biology 1999: 9, 665–671

(6) Jüttner M, Caelli T, Rentschler I: Evidence-based pattern classification: a structural approach to human perceptual learning and generalization. J Mathemat Psychol 1997: 41, 244–259

(7) Watanabe S: Pattern recognition. Human and mechanical. John Wiley & Sons, New York 1985

For further reading see a more detailed discussion of these issues by Rentschler I: Neuroaesthetic Theory of the Ugly Duckling. In: Noguchi K (ed): The psychology of Beauty and Kansei: New horizons of Gestalt Psychology. Fuzanbo International Publishers, Tokyo 2005

Senses and their Medialisation

MICHAEL METZELTIN, Professor of Romance languages

Senses and semiotic system

Cognition, ideas, contents of sentences, textuality man can transform into communication only via semiotics. Semiotics can be realized by our senses (touch, sight, equilibrium, hearing, smell, taste) only through perceptible media. Suitable perceptible media are: Body movements and positioning in space, voice, sounds and noises, drawings and pictures, building blocks and architectural structures, cosmetics, textiles and garments, gastronomic dishes. With the aid of body movements gesture language and pantomimic is created, with voice verbal language is formed, by sound patterns systems of musical notes. By drawings and pictures illustrations, pictograms and alphabets are born, with cosmetics textiles and clothing mode is formed and culinary creations result in the art of gastronomy. Essential characteristics of semiotics are, that, with their help we can reproduce something and combine constituents with one another. With the aid of such a codex of signs we can create semiotic products.

The primate of linguistic signs

Visibly more frequently as semiotic products are verbally realised texts. Verbal texts consist of words and sentences, display a recognisable beginning and a recognisable end and are focussed thematically. Their theme always points to a reference beyond the text. Thanks to their being analysable and the wide range of possible combinations, linguistic signs appear to be the most efficient semiotic means of man. They are built up by connections of certain sequences of sounds (words) with certain ideas to point to a certain reality. José Ortega y Gasset says in his Ensayo de estética a manera de prólogo (IV) that, one must separate three points in a linguistic expression, e.g., It hurts me: 1st the pain itself, which I feel, 2nd my imagination of this pain, which does not hurt by itself, 3rd the expression It hurts me. Frequently, it is easier to define the perceptible elements (the forms, the significants, the names, the lexemes) as much as the ideas expressed by the former (the contents, the significatives, the noemes) than are the signs of other codes.

Man addresses principally objects and assigns to them characteristics, conditions, processes, developments, actions. From this develop narratives, descriptions and arguments, from this textuality develops. The latter can be realised with various sign systems. It is obvious, however, that all non verbal semiotic products can be transformed into verbal texts. Pantomimic, painting, sculpture, architecture, music, generally are based on a narrative programme. A storm (Ludwig van Beethoven, 6th symphony), a victory (marches), a landscape (Charles Ives, Three Places in New England, Enrique Granados, Paisaje, Impromptus), an optimistic mood (Sergej Prokofjew, 5th symphony), can be the thematical basis of parcours musicaux. It is however possible to reach grade zero of narrativity with various media. This holds for orchestral music, abstract painting (Fernand Léger), certain types of lyric, cases where the virtuosity of form is in the foreground (ornamentalisation, virtuosity). Textuality apparently, seems to be the deeper basis of semiotic products, which may be more or less artificially, skilfully, artistically, textualised, transformed, pictured, filmed, sculptured, set in music.

Linguistic signs are the most efficient semiotic means of man but they do have their weaknesses and strengths in expressivity, as do all other media, as is apparent in a comparison of verbal narratives of creation, Michelangelo's Creation, Franz Joseph Haydn's oratory Die Schöpfung and the sculpture of the Swede Carl Milles Die Hand Gottes. Verbal texts can more easily express narrative sequence, painting and sculpture, narrative moments and descriptive quality, architecture the concept of space, theatre the frontal aspect of action, films the mobility. Informatics leads to increasing visualisation of signs and virtuality of semiotic signs, cp. Money becomes virtual. And virtual money is money which exists only electronically and serves as a substitute for cash.

Forms of mediality

Man is equipped multi-sensuously for his perceptions and it may be deducted that when communicating all senses should possibly employed and addressed. Semiotic products therefore should be conceived and executed principally according to this variety of senses.

In any ritual enaction of procedures important and universally valid for society, members will tend to utilize all available semiotic media. One may assume that such enactions will principally always be realised by pantomimic, by dance, music, words, pictures, scent, sculpture, architecture and gastronomy (as theatre performance, masses, churches, texts, symphonies, cycles of pictures, festive garments, banquets). These ritual performances seem to belong to the most original semiotic productions of all cultures and are, principally, targeted to all the senses.

Each society is determined by certain rites which mediate through all the senses a certain order governing the inter-human relations. Since these generally are transitions, the transformations entailed are coded by actions. The carriers of such actions can be static, descriptive, the actions themselves be illustrated by dynamics, narrative, or, especially by words . Rites mirror abstract relations of power transformed for better understanding by the audience into scenic narrations. Narrations can always be verbalised. Originating from such rites both textuality in general, and complex artistic œuvres developed. The desire for such an order becoming narrative, and a performance addressing all senses, appear to be a constant feature of anthropology.

By specialisation of actors, by the time, the entire complex of mediality is split up into various areas and a tendency to mono-mediality becomes manifest. By this token mono-medial objets d'art in architecture, sculpture, painting, pantomimic, dance, texts, pieces of music are created. It may be stated, that, if one medium is deleted, this may be compensated by multiplication of the action of another (re-medialisation). Michelangelo transferred to painted figures of the Sixtine Chapel categories of sculpture. The language of lyric, generally is strongly accented by musical and pictorial language thereby compensating for the lack of sound and sight: one may recall the stimuli of the poet Paul Verlaine De la musique avant toute chose and of musicality and richesse of illustrations, and more generally, the frequent use of synaesthesies of the Nicuagaran modernist Rubén Darío. The Mexican writer Laura Esquivel divides up her novel Como agua para chocolate (1989) into twelve chapters and assigns one month to each, with a fitting recipe, except for June where the (symbolic) recipe is the instruction for the making of matches.

The breaking up of a complex mediality and its transmission into a mono-mediality can be seen in context of a gradual secularisation of rites. Magical-religious parts of an originally ritual whole become pantomimic, dance, music, text, picture, sculpture, architecture, secularised forms of art devoid of their ritual character or stand just for themselves (l'art pour l'art), or, achieve a new meaning by a changing interpretation or context. Bereaved of their religious connection these mono-medialities form fields of scientific reflexion. One may think of, e.g., the Art poétique of Nicolas Boileau-Despréaux (1674) or the Investigaciones filosóficas sobre la belleza ideal considerada como objeto de todas las artes von Esteban Arteaga (1789), or the representatives of Russian formalism. Literature and life are separate and the literary oeuvre is subject to its own rules, whereby the formation of single disciplines and separation is enhanced and a comprehensive perspective is lost.

At the turn of the 16th century opera constitutes itself, as a narration of an (often) mythological character, a blend of verbal text, with ballet, music, ouverture, arias, recitatives and choir (viz. Claudio Monteverdi's Orfeo. Favola in musica, 1607). Also the Ballets de Cour at the court of Louis XIV, demonstrating the power of absolutism in an ideal world lead by France, tend to a multi-mediality (among other the Ballet des Nations as a supplement to Molière's Bourgeois gentilhomme, 1670: Le Temple de la Paix, 1685). At the end of the 18th century the interplay of the arts is again more intensively considered, a tendency which led Wagner to form the Gesamtkunstwerk. In the opera of the 19th century multimedia concept and intenseness of media coincide: not only different media are employed to illustrate the scene, the ways of expression of a singular medium takes up characteristics of another. Speech becomes musical, music produces a narrative. In the 20th century Jean-Louis Barrault (1910–1994) – Pantomime, Actor, Regisseur, Author – promotes the total theatre: Decoration, Light, Masks, Music, Noises (echos and accords) are important and equally essential constitutents of the scene. Theatre is enlivened by bringing onto the stage all measures of expression of man: Prose, lyric, song, cry, breathing, silence, symbolic and lyric gestures, dance. Films accentuate the multi-media expression of human narrative and re-interpretation of past opera (cp. A carta by Manuel de Oliveira and Eyes wide shut by Stanley Kubrick). Every-day communication, next to spoken words, consists widely of non verbal signs, such as gestures, mimic, looks, garments.

Thanks to the development of film, television, shows and internet we face an epoch where communication will happen rather in concert of all media, reconstructively, and lead to new visions of sense and context. We can differentiate today various forms of mediality:

Complex-mediality: all available media are employed for the expression of a performing œuvre
Pluri-mediality: several media are used for the purpose
Trans-mediality: an œuvre expressed by a particular medium is transposed into another (a special form of trans-mediality is the modernisation of opera)
Mono-mediality: only one medium is used for expression
Inter-mediality: a work produced by one medium points to another expressed in a different medium
Intra-mediality: a semiotic product of a collection (e.g. an album of songs) relates to another product of the same collection

Understanding and Visualisation

The methods for understanding semiotic products are always similar. For their understanding, an identification of its components is necessary (analysis) and thereby, the topic addressed can be recognized and their function elaborated (interpretation). The cognisance of narrative traits, of the description of persons and objects and of proofs is intended. This process is optimally achieved if the main topics of narration and description are expressed in complex mediality, especially visually. If a semiotic product tends to monomediality, the author must take care for better understanding of his œuvre and employ different ways of re-medialisation, e.g., visualisation of his text by metaphors or reference to pictures with similar themes, musicalisation of texts by combination of sounds and rhythms. He may also try to reconstitute the original complex mediality by reference to the activation of all senses.

An important role for the understanding of semiotic products play forms of repetition which amplify the textuality. The amplification not only creates coherence but permits identification of the main moments and elements. In Peter Iljitch Tchajkovskij's Swan Lake the figure of Odette is multiplied by her colleagues many times. This type of repetition makes it clear that what holds for the main role, in a lesser intensity also holds for all. A musical theme can be chiastically split and repeated in various tonality, with different instruments as by Alban Berg. Amplification results in redundancy necessary for communication.

A poet of re-medialisation: Baudelaire

Charles Baudelaire (1821-1867) is seen as the founder of poetical symbolism and modernité with his collections of Les fleurs du mal (1857) and Petits poèmes en prose (1869). He cultivates formal beauty and searches for the secret relation of matters. But he also was a critic and dealt with the works of Honoré Daumier, Eugène Delacroix, Édouard Manet. In his frequent descriptions of everyday life, of the morbidity of big cities, of evil and desire, it is evident that he relates to all possibilities of perception: time and again he relates to cris, risettes, glapissements, chants, caresses, regards, lumière, étincelles, senteurs, parfums, odeurs, sauts, danses. Objects frequently are étincelants. In Petite poème en prose XI he speaks of a woman «Dans sa rage, elle étincelle tout entière, comme le fer qu'on bat». All that glitters bring forward a secret symphony: «Les miroirs, les métaux, les étoffes, l'orfèvrerie, et la faïance y jouent pour les yeux une symphonie muette et mystérieuse» (XVIII). The poet even dreams of an infinity of perceptions «il est une contrée qui te ressemble, où tout est beau, riche, tranquille et honnête, où la fantaisie a bâti et décoré une Chine occidentale, où la vie est douce à respirer, où le bonheur est marié au silence. C'est là qu'il faut aller vivre, c'est là qu'il faut aller mourir! Oui, c'est là qu'il faut aller respirer, rêver et allonger les heures par l'infini des sensations» (Petits poèmes en prose, XVII, L'invitation au voyage).

Baudelaire's urge for visualisation

Next to the desire to write, Baudelaire seems to have had an urge for visual demonstration obvious also by his explicit dedication to painting. In Petit poème en prose XXXVI, carrying the title Le désir de peindre, he admits: «Je brûle de peindre celle qui m'est apparue si rarement et qui a fui si vite, comme une belle chose regrettable derrière le voyageur emporté dans la nuit.» And Petit poème en prose XXX reads how a painter relates the advantages of his profession: «Ma professions de peintre me pousse à regarder attentivement les visages, les physionomies, qui s'offrent dans ma route, et vous savez quelle jouissance nous tirons de cette faculté qui rend à nos yeux la vie plus vivante et plus significative que pour les autres hommes».

The sense of sight is ubiquitous in all the works of Baudelaire. Here we want to present the most important aspects of this sense, as registered by the poet in his Petit poèmes en prose.

Outwardly, the eyes, a look, may be dreadful, wonderful, inquisitive, big; rarely a colour is mentioned:

«Voilà bien ces yeux (sc. de l'Idole) dont la flamme traverse le crépuscule; ces subtiles et terribles mirettes (Augen), que je reconnais à leur effrayante malice!» (V)

«Je l'épiais (sc. une vieille affligée) longtemps pendant qu'elle cherchait dans les gazettes, avec des yeux actifs, jadis brûlés par les larmes, des nouvelles d'un intérêt puissant et personnel.» (XIII)

«Je ne puis jamais m'empêcher de jeter un regard, sinon universellement sympathique, au moins curieux, sur la foule de parias qui se pressent autour de l'enceinte d'un concert public.» (XIII)

«Pour moi, si je me penche vers la belle Féline, (...) au fond de ses yeux adorables je vois toujours l'heure distinctement, toujours la même, une heure vaste, solennelle, grande comme l'espace, sans division de minutes ni de secondes». (XIV)

«Je plongeais dans vos yeux si beaux et si bizarrement doux, dans vos yeux verts, habités par le Caprice et inspirés par la Lune» (XXVI)

«C'est en contemplant cette visiteuse que tes yeux se sont si bizarrement agrandis.» (XXXVII)

«Toutes ces fantasmagories sont presque aussi belles que les yeux de ma belle bien-aimée, la petite folle monstrueuse aux yeux verts.» (XLIV)

«C'était une grande fille, robuste, aux yeux très ouverts.» (XLVII)

Inwardly, the eyes may be seen as experienced, intensive, objective, professional, dark, mysterious:
«Un œil expérimenté ne s'y trompe jamais.» (XIII)

«Elle aussi, comme la plèbe à laquelle elle s'était mêlée et qu'elle ne voyait pas, elle regardait le monde lumineux avec un œil profond.» (XIII)

«Mais quel regard profond, inoubliable, il (le vieux saltimbanque) promenait sur la foule et les lumières, dont le flot mouvant s'arrêtait à quelques pas de sa répulsive misère!» (XIV)

«De l'autre côté de la grille, sur la route, entre les chardons et les orties, il y avait un autre enfant, sale, chétif, fuligineux, un des ces marmots-parias dont un œil impartial découvrirait la beauté, si, comme l'œil du connaisseur devine une peinture idéale sous un vernis de carrossier, il le nettoyait de la répugnante patine de la misère.» (XIX)

«Leurs grands yeux sombres sont devenus tout à fait brillants pendant qu'ils faisaient de la musique.» (XXXI)

«Ses yeux sont deux antres où scintille vaguement le mystére, et son regard illumine comme l'éclair.» (XXXVI)

The eye searches to understand, analyses, observes:
«Un de mes amis, le plus inoffensif rêveur qui ait existé, a mis une fois le feu à une forêt pour voir, disait-il, si le feu prenait avec autant de facilité qu'on l'affirme généralement.» (IX)

«Un autre allumera un cigare à côté d'un tonneau de poudre, pour voir, pour savoir, pour tenter la destinée.» (IX)

«Et, tout en analysant des yeux des détails de la gravure, il continuit mentalement.» (XXIV)

«Il y a une sorte de plaisir mystérieux et aristocratique pour celui qui n'a plus ni curiosité ni ambition, à contempler, couché dans le belvédère ou accoudé sur le môle, tous ces mouvements de ceux qui partent et de ceux qui reviennent, de ceux qui ont encore la force de vouloir, le désir de voyager ou de s'enrichir.» (XLI)

The eyes are able to express different moods: solitude, reserve, shame, disappointment, sadness, begging, idleness, dizziness, but also astonishment, ecstasy, desire, jealousy, hate, will and boldness or fraternity:
«Un de ces fous artificiels (...) lève des yeux pleins de larmes vers l'immortelle Déesse. Et ses yeux disent: – Je suis le dernier et le plus solitaire des humains». (VII)

«Un autre, timide à ce point qu'il baisse les yeux même devant les regards des hommes». (IX)

«Loin du regard insolent des joyeux et des oisifs». (XIII)

«Un œil expérimenté ne s'y trompe jamais. Dans ces traits rigides ou abattus, dans ces yeux caves et ternes, ou brillants des derniers éclairs de la lutte, dans ces rides profondes et nombreuses, dans ces démarches si lentes ou si saccadées, il déchiffre tout de suite les innombrables légendes de l'amour trompé (...)». (XIII)

«Il (le premier Satan) me regarda avec ses yeux inconsolablement navrés, d'où s'écoulait une insidieuse ivresse». (XXI)

«Ces six yeux contemplaient fixement le café nouveau (...). Les yeux du père disaient: ‚Que c'est beau! (...)' Les yeux du petit garçon: ‚Que c'est beau! mais c'est une maison où peuvent seuls entrer les gens qui ne sont pas comme nous'». (XXVI)

«Quant aux yeux du plus petit, ils étaient trop fascinés pour exprimer autre chose qu'une joie stupide et profonde». (XXVI)

«Ses yeux s' éclairaient d'un feu intérieur semblable à celui de la jalousie et de la rancune». (XXVII)

«Il y avait là des visages étranges d'hommes et de femmes, marqués d'une beauté fatale, qu'il me semblait avoir vus déjà à des époques et dans des pays dont il m'était impossible de me souvenir exactement». (XXIX)

«Nous vîmes, en approchant, que c'était une terre magnifique, éblouissante». (XXXIV)

In Petit poème en prose XLVII the poet points out that when walking in a city, various bizarre sights may be encountered as long as one is capable of looking.
«Quelles bizarreries ne trouve-t-on pas dans une grande ville quand on sait se promener et regarder?» (XLVII)

The eyes may have different effects with their looks: they may engulf, intimidate, cause delight:
«Voilà bien ces yeux (sc. de l'Idole) dont la flamme traverse le crépuscule; ces subtiles et terribles mirettes (eyes), que je reconnais à leur effrayante malice! Elles attirent, elles subjuguent, elles dévorent le regard de l'imprudent qui les contemple». (V)

«Ces gens-là me sont insupportables avec leurs yeux ouverts comme des portes cochères». (XXVI)

«Chacun s'abandonna, sans inquiétude, aux voluptés multipliées que donne la vue d'un chef-d'œuvre d'art vivant». (XXVII)

«Le commissaire (...) me regarda de travers (...) mû sans doute par un désir invétéré et une habitude d'état de faire peur». (XXX)

«Ses yeux sont deux antres où scintille vaguement le mystère, et son regard illumine comme l'éclair». (XXXVI)

«Il ya a des femmes qui inspirent l'envie de les vaincre et de jouir d'elles; mais celle-ci donne le désir de mourir lentement sous son regard». (XXXVI)

«J'ai connu une certaine Bénédicta, qui remplissait l'atmosphère d'idéal, et dont les yeux répandaient le désir de la grandeur, de la beauté, de la gloire et de tout ce qui fait croire à l'immortalité». (XXXVIII)

Baudelaire as a master of re-medialisation

In the introduction to his Petits poèmes en prose Baudelaire expresses his wish to write a musical prose corresponding to particular moods:
«Quel est celui de nous qui n'a pas, dans ses jours d'ambition, rêvé le miracle d'une prose poétique, musicale sans rythme et sans rime, assez souple et assez heurtée pour s'adapter aux mouvements lyriques de l'âme, aux ondulations de la rêverie, aux soubresauts de la conscience?» (À Arsène Houssaye)

In Petit poèmes en prose III (Le confiteor de l'artiste) he emphasizes the importance of musicality and visualisation in poetry:
«Grand délice que celui de noyer son regard dans l'immensité du ciel et de la mer! Solitude, silence, incomparable chasteté de l'azur! une petite voile frissonnante à l'horizon, et qui par sa petitesse et son isolement imite mon irrémédiable existence, mélodie monotone de la houle, toutes ces choses pensent par moi, ou je pense par elles (car dans la grandeur de la rêverie, le moi se perd vite!); elles pensent, dis-je, mais musicalement et pittoresquement, sans arguties, sans syllogismes, sans déductions».

Despite the fact that Baudelaire writes "only" texts he always attempts to instill into those the highest possible musicality and visuality but also activate all senses. This he achieves by employment of various means of re-medialisation. As an example the following poem may serve: XVII Un Hémisphère dans une Chevelure (loc.cit., ed. Robert Kopp, Gallimard 1973):

Laisse-moi respirer longtemps, longtemps, l'odeur
de tes cheveux, y plonger tout mon visage, comme
un homme altéré dans l'eau d'une source, et les
agiter avec ma main comme un mouchoir odorant,
pour secouer des souvenirs dans l'air.
Si tu pouvais savoir tout ce que je vois! tout ce
que je sens! tous ce que j'entends dans tes cheveux!
Mon âme voyage sur le parfum comme l'âme
des autres hommes sur la musique.
Tes cheveux contiennent tout un rêve, plein de
voilures et de mâtures; ils contiennent de grandes
mers dont les moussons me portent vers de char-
mants climats, où l'espace est plus beau et plus
profond, où l'atmosphère est parfumée par les
fruits, par les feuilles et par la peau humaine.
Dans l'océan de ta chevelure, j'entrevois un port
fourmillant de chants mélancoliques, d'hommes
vigoureux de toutes nations et de navires de toutes
formes découpant leurs architectures fines et compli-
quées sur un ciel immense où se prélasse l'éternelle
chaleur.
Dans les caresses de ta chevelure, je retrouve les
langueurs des longues heures passées sur un divan,
dans la chambre d'un beau navire, bercées par le
roulis imperceptible du port, entre les pots de
fleurs et les gargoulettes rafraîchissantes.
Dans l'ardent foyer de ta chevelure, je respire
l'odeur du tabac mêlé à l'opium et au sucre; dans
la nuit de ta chevelure, je vois resplendir l'infini de

l’azur tropical; sur les rivages duvetés de ta chevelure je m’enivre des odeurs combinées du goudron, du musc et de l’huile de coco.

Laisse-moi mordre longtemps tes tresses lourdes et noires. Quand je mordille tes cheveux élastiques et rebelles, il me semble que je mange des souvenirs.

The theme of the text is a certain type of hair of a woman which is likened to a hemisphere/ it is reminiscent of an hemisphere (a semi-globe, half-a-world is called up as a vision; cf. title, subject and direct objects, semantic repetitions). The contents of the text is visually rounded as the first and last paragraphs, by repetition of Laissez moi and of souvenir, form so to say a “loop”:

Careful and loud reading reveals a series of obvious repetitions which amplify the text and at the same time confer cohesion:

Phonetic repetitions: Laisse-moi … longtemps, longtemps, l’odeur (1), les langueurs des longues heures (23), Laisse-moi … longtemps … lourdes (33) (repetition of liquida evokes the imagination of flowing and the noise of water/waves, regular and rhythmic wavy movements), // chevelure (title, 1, 16, 17, 27, 30–31), voilures et de mâtures (11) (repetition of the vowel ü represents the idea of “pulling out”).

Anapher: dans tes cheveux (7), Dans l’océan de ta chevelure (16), Dans les caresses de ta chevelure (22), dans la chambre d’un beau navire (24), Dans l’ardent foyer de ta chevelure (37), dans la nuit de ta chevelure (28–29). (The anaphoric repetition of the locative preposition “dans” contributes to visualise a certain locus, here, the rich hair.)
Semantic field: Mon âme voyage (8), plein de voilures et de mâtures (10–11), de grandes mers dont les moussons me portent vers de charmants climats (11–13), l’océan (16), un port (16), navires (18), navire (24), port (25), rivages (30) (These words point to the idea and the imagination of “travel”) // odeur (1), parfum (8), parfumée par les fruits, par les feuilles et par la peau humaine (14–15), fleurs (26), l’odeur du tabac mêlé à l’opium et au sucre (28), des odeurs combinées du goudron, du musc et de l’huile de coco (31–32) (Repetition of the reference to odours intends to let these emerge in phantasy.)
The senses are activated also by various allusions of the poet:
Sensing in general: tout ce que je sens (6–7)
Touch: y (= les cheveux) plonger tout mon visage (2), les (= cheveux) agiter avec ma main (3–4), l’éternelle chaleur (20–21), les caresses de ta chevelure (22), l’ardent foyer de ta chaleur (27), les rivages duvetés de ta chevelure (31–32)

Sight: tout ce que je vois (6), j’entrevois un port fourmillant de chants mélancoliques (16–17), je vois resplendir l’infini de l’azur tropical (29–30)

Equilibrium: bercées par le roulis imperceptible du port (24–25)

Hearing: tout ce que j'entends dans tes cheveux (8), comme l'âme des autres hommes voyage sur la musique (8–9), j'entrevois un port fourmillant de chants mélancoliques (16-17)
Smell: respirer ... l'odeur de tes cheveux (1–2), mon âme voyage sur le parfum (8), l'atmosphère est parfumée par les fruits, par les feuilles et par la peau humaine (15–16), je respire l'odeur du tabac mêlé à l'opium et au sucre (27–28), je m'enivre des odeurs combinées du goudron, du musc et de l'huile de coco (31-32)

Touch: les gargoulettes rafraîchissantes (26), mordre ... tes tresses (33), je mordille tes cheveux (34), je mange (35)

Another form of re-medialisation points to various media:
Body movements, positioning in space: y plonger tout mon visage (2), les agiter avec ma main (2–4), les caresses (22) (leading to an imagination of love)

Voice, sounds, noises: la musique (9), chants mélancoliques (17) (> mood)

Drawings, pictures: l'espace est plus bleu et plus profond (13–14), je vois resplendir l'infini de l'azur tropical (29–30) (> remoteness)

Building blocks, constructions: plein de voilures et de mâtures (10–11), navires ... découpant leurs architectures fines et compliquées (18–20), dans la chambre d'un beau navire (24) (> distance)

Cosmetics, textiles, garments: le parfum (8), l'odeur (28), odeurs (31) (> inebriation)

A rhetoric commentary of titles an paragraphs shows how the poet utilises all means to make the reader transform in his phantasy the text into a multi-media scenario:

Title: the metonym 'hair' > 'upper part of the head', provokes comparison 'hair' = 'hemisphere', and by the aid of dimensional incongruence the whole wide world arises).

Paragraph 1: The imperative at the beginning laisse-moi points to an activity which, by repetition in the last paragraph, should last till then. The adverb longtemps underlines that. The first direct object odeur relates to the importance of the olfactory sense. Hair is compared to water (the Ego needs hair as it needs water), on the other hand a handkerchief is taken for allusion, with the aid of which the ego disperses memories (souvenirs), repeated in the last strophe and which, together with the hair make up one theme. The ego caresses the hair of a You and so recalls certain memories.

Paragraph 2: The three exclamatory sentences reflect the inner swell of emotions of the Ego in which three senses partake. The triplicate mention of tout relates to the great dimension which is captured by the senses. The fragrance of hair let the Ego travel.

Paragraph 3: The travel is a dream made with ships and monsoon winds leading to distant oceans and ports in the Far East. Charmants climats and l'espace est plus bleu et plus profond point to a world perceived in a special way, principally by smell as clearly evidenced in the description où l'atmosphère est parfumée par les fruits, par les feuilles et par la peau humaine.

Paragraph 4: The chevelure, a source in paragraph 1 and the sea in paragraph 3, now turns into an ocean, the imagined harbour is filled with songs, people and ships, the sky is beyond measure and the heat eternal: the dream world where the Ego arrived has no borders.

Paragraph 5: In this dream world the Ego meets again the longing and melancholy (indicated by the onomatopoeia of the sound l).

Paragraph 6: The source (well) now became a foyer (hearth), the Ego breathes a mixture of tobacco, opium, and sugar, of tar, musk and coconut oil, becomes inebriated and watches blue infinity, has become limitless.

Paragraph 7: The Ego always wants to bite the hair, thereby however it eats up all its memories and terminates the inebriation.

While the title permits to expect a description, the poet delineates a trance process, which is re-medialised by many allusions to sensory perceptions:

To inhale the fragrance of hair (1) > a new dimension of sight, feeling and hearing (2) > All appears distant, enchanting, more blue, deeper (3) > All appears infinite (4) > a certain langueur is once again reached (5) > inebriation (6) > sobriety (7).
In hindsight the poem can be interpreted biographically (one consider the relation of the poet to Jeanne Duval, who was painted by Edouard Manet, and one compare the description of the woman as a "soleil noir" in poem XXXVI Le désir de peindre) or more generally, when such emotions are re-enacted.

Re-medialisation can be enhanced if intra-mediality, trans-mediality and inter-mediality are taken into consideration:

Intra-mediality: chevelure is metioned and described also in other Petits poèmes en prose: «Le poids de son énorme chevelure presque bleue tire en arrière sa tête délicate et lui donne un air triomphant et paresseux». (XXV, La belle Dorothée)
«Le temps n'a rien arraché de son abondante crinière d'où s'exhale en fauves parfums toute la vitalité endiablée du Midi français: Nîmes, Aix, Arles, Avignon, Narbonne, Toulouse, villes bénies du soleil, amoureuses et charmantes». (XXXIX, Un cheval de race)

Trans-mediality: Un Hémisphère dans une Chevelure dates from 1857. In 1859 Baudelaire wrote a rhymed version (La Chevelure).

Inter-mediality: Our text is reminiscent of other poems in various languages and from different epochs which do address hair as a topic (viz. several poems of the Italian Giambattista Marino (1569–1625) or Suelta al céfiro blando by the Spaniard Esteban Manuel de Villegas (1589–1669). The description of hair plays an important role in the Song of Songs. Amongst the contemporaries and followers of Baudelaire the poem La Chevelure by Pierre Louys (1870–1925) may be pointed out, also the poem La fille aux cheveux de lin von Charles-Marie Leconte de Lisle (1818–1894) (music by Claude Debussy). The long hair of a woman is again a frequent topic in painting, e.g. Fischblut by Gustav Klimt, illustration for Apuleius by Charles Ricketts.

If one compares all these presentations in various media, it seems that a (masculine) archetype is created: typical characteristic of such a woman is, having long, wavy hair which is likened to streaming water; such hair is smooth, flexible, therefore attractive, such hair is bewitching and captures the man, leads him into special worlds and transmits particular messages. Or, more poetically worded:

«Des rêves! toujours des rêves! et plus l'âme est ambitieuse et délicate, plus les rêves l'éloignent du possible. Chaque homme porte en lui sa dose d'opium naturel, incessamment sécrétée et renouvelée, et, de la naissance à la mort, combien comptons-nous d'heures remplies par la jouissance positive, par l'action réussie et décidée? Vivrons-nous jamais, passerons-nous jamais dans ce tableau qu'a peint mon esprit, ce tableau qui te ressemble»?

«Ces trésors, ces meubles, ce luxe, cet ordre, ces parfums, ces fleurs miraculeuses, c'est toi. C'est encore toi, ces grands fleuves et ces canaux tranquilles. Ces énormes navires qu'ils charrient, tout chargés de richesses, et d'où montent les chants monotones de la manœuvre, ce sont mes pensées qui dorment ou qui roulent sur ton sein. Tu les conduis doucement vers la mer qui est l'Infini, tout en réfléchissant les profondeurs du ciel dans la limpidité de ta belle âme; – et quand, fatigués par la houle et gorgés de produits de l'Orient, ils rentrent au port natal, ce sont encore mes pensées enrichies qui reviennent de l'Infini vers toi». (XVIII, L'Invitation au Voyage).

True to Nature: Ethics of Medical Imagery

Stella Fatović-Ferenčić and Karl Holubar

In medicine, the transition from a text based to a picture dependent field developed slowly from the 16th century onwards. Before the advent of photography, other means of illustration were en vogue and, ever more often, included in printed texts. The atmosphere of scientific asceticism of the 19th century created the urge of a true to nature objectivity also in medical imaging. Furthermore the imperative true to nature stimulated tendencies in imaging which focused on extraordinary features, rare malformations and breathtaking disfigurations. By the beginning of the 20th century there was hardly a medical discipline which expressed itself without visual aids. Continuous increment of imaging in education and medicine parallels a process of alienation throughout the 20th century. One is tempted to speculate about the interdependency of these two phenomena. Furthermore medical imaging is rapidly moving beyond the sphere of medicine and conquers the public through different media. Anatomy, pathology and lately forensic medicine became part of our everyday life and it seems that the desire for it is as keen as the one for fashion models. Consequently there are estimations which suggest caution to the excessive use of pictures in science(1) as well as those which have little scientific and educational value(2). And Sonntag's analysis explored the response to images of horror and concluded that pictures may instill apathy and foster violence in observers(3).

Working in medical iconography(4), questions crept up in our minds, when sifting through piles of historical illustrations prints, drawings, gouaches, water colours, preserved in the vaults of the Institute for the History of Medicine in Vienna. After looking at all the many different kinds of pictures and after perusing the related notes from yesteryear, there was one which attracted our particular attention and we decided to single it out. The picture is a copper print, undated and unsigned, but surely from late 18th or early 19th century(5). In our perception, this image differed markedly from the rest of the illustrations because it evoked powerful feelings in the observer and provoked questions, what the particular message to be conveyed should be, by the artist or the employer. We felt challenged to inquire as to the borders between didactic medical imaging, and voyeuristic perversity, scientific idealism and sensationalism of the lay world.

The picture presents the head of a woman, cut off and displayed on a plate looking like the head of John the Baptist in art galleries. The legend reads that it is the head of a syphilitic prostitute who died in 1796, in an asylum, close to today's premises in Vienna.

Why this picture was collected in our files, and as a separate copy included in an album of paintings from the 18th and 19th centuries, is unknown. Contrary to all other images, this one aims at conferring a much broader message. It seems that a prostitute was not considered suitable to teach clinical manifestations of disease as were the others images. She should pose a threat and warning. A grotesque face, few teeth in mouth, the eyes sunken back into the orbitae, - an overall disfigured somehow animalistic image. A paradigma, accentuating how easily beauty turns into ruin, and how dreadful punishment for sins can be. The artist succeeded in attracting the attention of the beholder as much as instilling the image deep into the observer's memory. One can't resist to think that a sadistic attitude was operative. To shock, was the purpose of this image at the end of the 18th century, and shocking and exaggeration is the purpose of many of the pictures in the media-world of today. The only difference is that images which were of scientific importance only, in the past, are presented ever more frequently to the public today.

The citizen of the 21st century gets the impression, that the preservation and presentation of such an object, its selection for being portrayed by the authorities of then, moves us into a shadowy area where pathology, society, statal omnipotence and individual perversity border each other or overlap. Be it a head decapitated in the autopsy room, or the head of a juridically executed criminal, fried corpses, collections of hymenes, all violate taste as much as humanity, and are a sign of a morbid society. Even if it is, at times, only a literary phenomenon, as, e.g., Herzmanovsky-Orlando' s black humor, when Eynhuf, collects deciduous teeth of virgins to make a necklace(6). Also, one is tempted to recall henchmen's defiant reports(7) of the final moments of hanged criminals, during which the culprits experience lustful sensations and a terminal ejaculation. Again a sadistic attitude may be surmised, so to say, "it can't be that bad, after all, to end on the gallows".

The history of syphilis and other venerea, leprosy, vitiligo, lupus vulgaris, reveals examples of stigmatization and ostracision, by ignorant and powerful authorities and by a bigot society. Educated people from academia are no exception, viz. the Tuskegee syphilis study. And above all, on an enormous and blatantly criminal scale, the experiments of the Nazi era. This depictured head of a syphilitic woman stands almost symbolically for all victims, prostitutes, insane, malformed, poor, - all marginalized subpopulations which were not only cut off from society during their lifetime but denied humane treatment even after death. One suspects, they were used also for intimidation, and additionally, created a discrediting whiff of sensation when presented in museums and in curiosity cabinets. Many of such objects have been removed already from display.

Certainly, more respect is needed, also in medicine and its museums, contrary to what the sensationalism of the media-world insinuates by sprinkling the globe with every accessible drop of blood. In fact, in many instances, words may suffice, images are not needed. Anatomy/pathology, has been so beautifully exercised by our ancestors and later in various collections that are educative as much as ravishingly attractive to the eye of the beholder, medical and lay persons alike (Fig.74). Such objects should antagonize modern attempts to create a "real" world of human anatomy/pathology as recently presented in a giant and grisly exposition. True to nature was our aim from the 18th century on. We spoiled it in turning it into a grotesque picture-world. Iconography in medicine, of pain, of sickness and stigmatisation as well as our lack of respect and concern is no doubt true to nature- our modern nature, violent, hungry for horror and sensation, and not sensitive enough to suffering.

In the President's Message[8] of Carol Black, president of the Royal College of Physicians, it reads, "the reformed GMC (General Medical Council) asked the Colleges to prepare statements of standards against which doctors can assess their own performance." Yes, this is what we need, assess our own performance, not only working with our patients but also sticking to standards of imaging when we move from bedside to museum or stage exhibitions. Underpinning this objective of countenance, we refrain from presenting an illustration of the head in question.

References

(1) Ottino JM: Is a picture worth 1000 words? Exciting new illustration technologies should be used with care. Nature 2003; 421: 474-476
(2) Korf H-W, Wicht H: The public cadaver. Nature 2004; 428:805
(3) Sonntag S: Regarding the Pain of the Others. Penguin, London, 2003
(4) Fatović-Ferenčić, S Plewig G, Holubar K: Skin in Water-colours. Blackwell, Berlin, 2003
(5) Lesky E: Meilensteine der Wiener Medizin. Maudrich, Wien 1981
(6) Herzmanovsky-Orlando F v: Der Gaulschreck im Rosennetz. In: Das Gesamtwerk, (Torberg F ed). Langen-Müller, München 1963
(7) Lang J: Die Erinnerungen des österreichischen Scharfrichters, (Seyerl H ed). Seyerl, Wien 1996
(8) Black C: President's Message. Royal College of Physicians, College Commentary, January/February 2005

Why then a book on iconography?
Paraphrase: "and what is the use of a book without pictures" (L Caroll, Alice)

The factual availability of hidden or unknown historical originals
We wanted to design a (literary) experiment where the modern physician is confronted with historical imagery and stimulated to draw his own conclusions, also as to the relation of painted versus digital images.
The demonstration of artistic talent by medical doctors, professors even, witnessing the emphasis given to those faculties in the past. The educational proximity of the sciences to the humanities is evidenced thereby, a proximity we lack in our present-day educational curricula. Howard Spiro wrote "... literature and art are the wellsprings of empathy"* This we should keep in mind.
We, the principal authors of this book, different by gender, age, specialty, language, temper, would wish that our elaboration will, demonstrate how well, perhaps how much better, our ancestors were able to depict and highlight disease, and stimulate study of the past, of the humanities (literature, music etc.) and eventually proselytize for a more comprehensive self education, one beyond statistics and antigens.

The humanities have been moved to backstage in medical education, given the difficulty to accommodate all the modern sub-disciplines into the curriculum. A great difficulty, indeed. Modern medicine with informed consent, and with forced upon - (the patient) - information about every nook of the body and what's going on there, has shifted most of the load anyone of these "results" may confer, from the doctor to the patient. And the latter is left alone, with NMR shadows, X-ray images, fancy acronyms and more often than not, devoid of sufficient guidance, of empathy, of compassion. Only years of life lived, and dedication to the humanities, will enable us to cope with this dilemma.

* Spiro HM: Empathy and the Practice of Medicine. Beyond pills and the scalpel. Yale University Press 1993, p.133 ff.

Index of Contributors and Principal Authors

Abel
Abel Jan Odorich MD
Ophthalmologist
Baden, Austria
Dr.Abel@mycity.at

Aberer
Werner Aberer MD
Professor of Dermatology
Department of Dermatology
Division of Environmental Dermatology
Medical University of Graz
Graz, Austria
werner.aberer@klinikum-graz.at

Amm
Marita Amm MD
Martin-Luther-University Halle-Wittenberg
Department of Ophthalmology
Halle / Saale, Germany
marita.amm@medizin.uni-halle.de

Denk
Helmut Denk MD FRCPath
Professor and Chairman
Department of Pathology
Medical University of Graz
Graz, Austria
helmut.denk@meduni-graz.a

Druml
Wilfred Druml MD
Professor of Medicine
Medical University of Vienna
Vienna, Austria
wilfred.druml@meduniwien.ac.at

Fatović-Ferenčić
Stella Fatović-Ferenčić MD PhD
Professor of History of Medicine
Croatian Academy of Sciences and Arts
Department for History and Philosophy of Science
Division for History of Medical Science
Zagreb, Croatia,
stella@hazu.hr

Grabner
Günther Grabner MD
Professor and Chairman
Department of Ophthalmology
Paracelsus Medical University
Salzburg, Austria
g.grabner@salk.at

Happle
Rudolf Happle MD
Professor of Dermatology
Department of Dermatolgy
Philipp University of Marburg
Marburg, Germany
happle@med.uni-marburg.de

Holubar
Karl Holubar MD FRCP GSE
Professor of History of Medicine and of Dermatology, the Max and Margareta Wolf Library for the History of Dermatology
Institute for the History of Medicine
Center of Public Health
Medical University of Vienna
Vienna, Austria
karl.holubar@meduniwien.ac.at

Jaeger
Edward A. Jaeger MD
Professor of Ophthalmology
Jefferson Medical College of Thomas Jefferson University and
Attending Surgeon, Wills Eye Hospital
Philadelphia, Pennsylvania, U.S.A.
EYEBALLONE@aol.com

Jellinger
Kurt A. Jellinger MD
Professor of Neurology and Neuropatholoy
Institute of Clinical Neurobiology
Medical University of Vienna
Vienna, Austria
kurt.jellinger@univie.ac.at

Kampik
Anselm Kampik MD FEBO
Professor and Chairman
Department of Ophthalmology
Ludwig Maximilian University
Munich, Germany
anselm.kampik@med.uni-muenchen.de

Metzeltin
Michael Metzeltin PhD Prof hon
Professor and Chairman
Department of Romance Languages
University of Vienna,
Vienna, Austria
michael.metzeltin@univie.ac.at

Nussenblatt
Robert B. Nussenblatt MD
Chief, Laboratory of Immunology
National Eye Institute, National Institutes of Health
Bethesda, Maryland, USA
Dr.Bob@NEI.NIH.GOV

Ohara
Kuniaki Ohara MD
Professor and Chairman
Toranomon Hospital
Tokyo, Japan
k.ohara@toranomon.gr.jp

Plewig
Gerd Plewig MD MD hon FRCP
Professor and Chairman
Department of Dermatology
Luwig Maximilian University
Munich, Germany
gerd.plewig@med.uni-muenchen.de

Propping
Peter Propping, MD
Professor and Chairman
Institute of Human Genetics
Rheinische Friedrich Wilhelms University
Bonn, Germany
propping@uni-bonn.de

Rentschler
Ingo Rentschler PhD
Professor, Institute of Medical Psychology
Ludwig Maximilian University
Munich, Germany
ingo.rentschler@lrz.uni-muenchen.de

Shelley
Walter B Shelley MD PhD MACP
Professor Emeritus of Dermatology
Medical University of Ohio
Toledo OH USA
wshelley@meduohio.edu

Slezak
Hans Slezak MD
Professor and Chairman emeritus
Department of Ophthalmology
Medical University of Vienna
Vienna, Austria

Stingl
Georg Stingl MD MD hon
Professsor and Chairman
Division of Immunology, Allergy and Infectious Diseases
Department of Dermatology
Medical University of Vienna
Vienna, Austria
georg.stingl@meduniwien.ac.at

Tonn
Joerg-Christian Tonn MD
Professor and Chairman
Department of Neurosurgery
Ludwig Maximilian University
Munich, Germany
joerg.christian.tonn@med.uni-muenchen.de

Wilkinson
Darrell Wilkinson MD
Consultant Dermatologist retired
Amersham, Bucks. HP6 5HT
England, UK